HERE & NOW

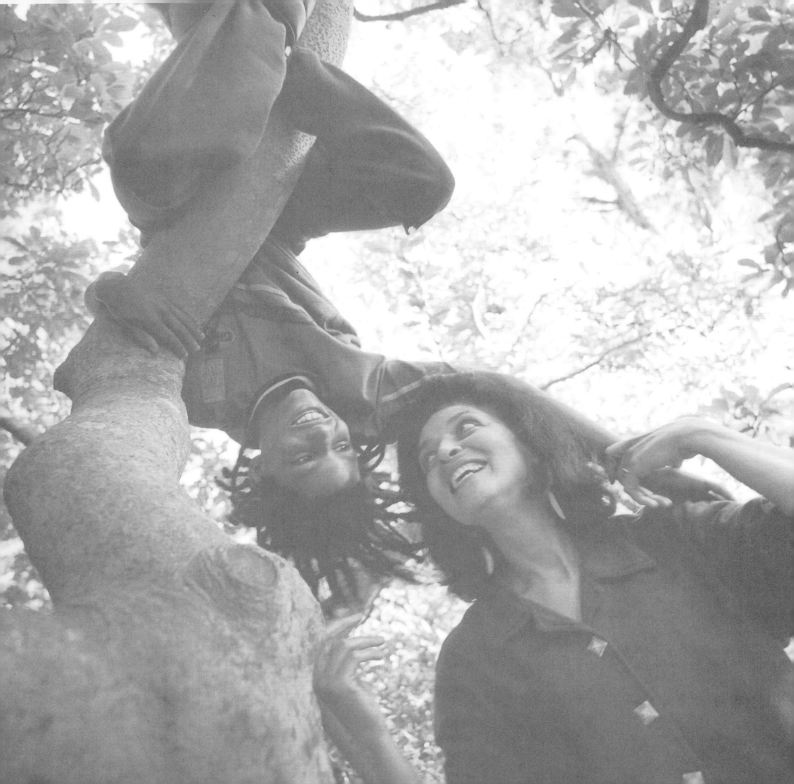

ELENA DORFMAN AND
HEIDI SCHULTZ ADAMS

Photographs by Elena Dorfman

INSPIRING STORIES OF
CANCER SURVIVORS

HERE & NOW

MARLOWE & COMPANY ■ NEW YORK

HERE AND NOW: *Inspiring Stories of Cancer Survivors*

Copyright © 2002 by Elena Dorfman and Heidi Schultz Adams

Photographs copyright © 2002 by Elena Dorfman

Published by

Marlowe & Company

An Imprint of Avalon Publishing Group

161 William Street, 16th Floor

New York, NY 10038

Library of Congress Cataloging-in-Publication Data is available for this title.

ISBN 1-56924-603-3

9   8   7   6   5   4   3   2   1

Designed by Pauline Neuwirth, Neuwirth and Associates, Inc.

Printed in the United States of America

Distributed by Publishers Group West

For Dave Marsh and Barbara Carr,

who started the whole thing years ago in their kitchen,

and for all of you whose lives have been touched by cancer.

 A PORTION OF THE PROCEEDS OF THIS BOOK
WILL BE DONATED TO PLANET CANCER.

Contents

■

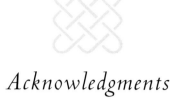

Acknowledgments

■

OUR DEEPEST THANKS to all of the amazing people who opened their hearts and shared their stories with us. We'd like to thank our agent, Sandy Choron, who believed. Our editor, Matthew Lore, because he never once yelled at us for missing deadlines when we had to talk to "just one more person." Lee and Daniel, your patience knows no bounds. Nelda, you didn't want to be singled out so we're thanking your fingers, which fly over a keyboard faster than ten speeding bullets.

This book would not have come to life without the help of: Ken Schultz, Chad Schultz, Chris Schultz, Tasha Greiling, Karen Swymer, Marlo Thomas, M.P. Nourzad and Team NourzAds, the Wellness Center at Newton Center, Harry Choron, Eileen Manela, Ilyse Gordon, David Rowan, Jennifer Rowan, Ken Torres, Olivia Rowan, Neil Elder, Dr. Ian Zlotlow, Michael Solomon, Vivek Tiwary, Dylan Schaffer, Ava and Susan Abromowitz and Mouna, Dr. Bob Mennel, Dr. Wynne Snoots and his Flurry-loving staff, Miriam Baum, Noel "Juiceman" Brohner, Carol and Gerry Abrams, Adrienne Levin, Gail Brohner, Marty Nessum, the Wellness Center at Woodland Hills, Anne Fitzsimons, Amgen and their Courage Awards program, Gail Dorfman, Mr. Wendy Earl, Yvo Riezebos, Jon Polk, and all the other people without whom this book would not have come together—you know who you are.

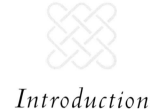

Introduction

Why Another Cancer Book?

*T*YPE "CANCER BOOK" into an online search engine and it returns more than a million matches. Books to guide patients through the experience. Books from every imaginable perspective: traditional, alternative, personal, medical, nutritional, spiritual. These resources are indispensable, if you're sick. But what happens *after*?

When we met, Elena was fifteen years out of treatment; Heidi, seven—far from the time when weeks were measured by the slow drip of an IV. Despite the profusion of cancer guides, we found little that addressed our needs and concerns as survivors.

Having cancer was, for us both, an exceptional, momentous experience. It was the marker against which we measured time, the looking glass through which we watched our lives. And then, one day, it wasn't. We had made it through, each in our own way. And over time, we grew curious to see how everyone else had made it.

We learned that for some, cancer is just an interruption—life returns to normal with scarcely a backwards glance. For others, a diagnosis leads to drastic life changes.

That we've been out of treatment so long does not make us medical exceptions. There are more than ten million people living today who have a history of cancer. More and more people are questioning what happens when treatment ends. More and more people are talking about what it means to survive a life-threatening illness.

We wanted to explore the difference cancer had made in people's lives. And in the process of asking others these questions, we hoped to gain a deeper understanding of our own experiences, so many years later.

Where We Are, Here and Now

ELENA DORFMAN

THIS PROJECT IS my epilogue to rhabdomyosarcoma, the disease which, since I was sixteen, has been the book of my days.

Prologue: I was a junior in high school. Skateboards, clothes, cars. Summer nights hopping from pool to pool, boy to boy, one adolescent drama to another. And then the lump on my wrist, which could have been tendonitis, which might have been benign, dragged me kicking and screaming out of my teenage bubble and into an alien, terrifying world.

The story begins: What else is there to say? I threw up for two years. And then my mom died of breast cancer, which did not improve the experience.

When I finally emerged from a fog of applesauce and Cytoxan, I realized I'd been remarkably lonely during treatment. I knew almost no one my age who had the slightest idea of what I was talking about, what I had been through, what it meant to have cancer. I had so many questions: Am I too sad? Am I attractive? Do I tell people? Answers of one sort or another came, slowly, through the lens of an old camera my dad gave me.

I took pictures, thousands of pictures of people like me. And what emerged was a book called *The C-Word: Teenagers and their Families Living With Cancer.* I wanted to give them a mirror. I wanted them to be able to open a book and know they were not alone.

Several chapters ahead: After years of thinking about and talking about what it means to have cancer at sixteen—to kids and medical professionals around the country—I was suddenly an adult. My identification with the disease began to fade. I was considered, by all accounts, cured. Living in California, working as a commercial photographer, I became, over time, separate from the characters and settings that had defined my illness. Now, nearly two decades after diagnosis, the deep connections have dissipated. I have to fight sometimes to keep the lessons in mind.

Working on this project, working with Heidi, taking pictures of these extraordinary people—it's a reminder, a trip back. It's an end of sorts too, a goodbye. I'd be lying if I said I wasn't happy to leave cancer behind. It is a story filled with remarkable characters. It compelled me to shun the easy choices, the mediocre experiences. It taught me to fight, to be vulnerable, empathetic, better, always better. It made me restless, quick to the essence of things, impatient with the unnecessary. It left Post-It notes everywhere: "Think Elena"; "Be Conscious"; "The Clock's Ticking, What Are You Waiting For?" Its constant alarm made me a little crazy, for sure, but it enriched my life beyond description. I'll thank my book of rhabdomyosarcoma as I gently lay it down.

So this is it: My postscript to cancer. I can't imagine what my life would look like without it. And I wouldn't want to know.

HEIDI SCHULTZ ADAMS

ASIDE FROM THE obvious explanation, there's a more subtle, but perhaps more important reason that cancer brought me to this book: it was cancer that gave me the courage to call myself a writer. Or maybe "courage" is the wrong word: cancer took away my excuses.

I won't invoke that perplexing refrain, "Cancer is the best thing that ever happened to me." I just can't say that, having endured the devastation and terrible irony of losing people I loved to the same disease I survived. However, I will say that cancer altered the direction of my life such that I haven't the faintest idea who I would be today without it.

I left home for college at sixteen, anxious to get a head start on "real life." After graduating, I did what all self-respecting English majors do: I hit the road. I tended bar in London, started smoking, worked in a Parisian brokerage firm, sunbathed topless, hiked the Grand Canyon, stopped smoking. I was on an enjoyable journey, but one with no real direction beyond accumulating dazzling journal entries—which I was too insecure to show anyone. An essential element was missing from my life, but I couldn't put my finger on it.

At twenty-six, I began experiencing excruciating pain in my left ankle; pain that jolted me awake, night after night. Finally one day, after months of misdiagnoses, the words "Ewing's sarcoma" were permanently seared into my brain. I had bone cancer.

Before my diagnosis, I approached experiences as an observer, keeping them at arm's length with pen and paper, rather than being truly absorbed and affected. This time, I committed. I plunged so deeply into the experience that it brutally shoved me off the sidelines of my life and into the fray, no holds barred.

After my treatment ended, I was completely hairless, bone-weary—and ready to take on the world. A year and a half of battling insurance companies, questioning doctors and enduring double-takes at my shiny baldness had toughened me. I no longer feared criticism. I didn't have to be perfect. And in facing down a life-threatening illness, I had discovered the missing essential element in my life: taking a stake in it.

And that changed everything.

Once cancer had shown me what I was capable of, I couldn't fall back on the easy stuff, avoiding what I *really* wanted to do because it might be risky or difficult. The fact that I might fail, that I might be less than perfect, was no longer an excuse for not trying. So I took a deep breath and started writing for a living, working as a magazine editor, freelance writer and ad copywriter. I founded Planet Cancer [www.planetcancer.org], a non-profit organization that helps young adults with cancer support each other—my personal stand against the isolation I had felt during my treatment.

When Elena invited me to undertake this book with her, it took me approximately a nanosecond to give a resounding "yes." I had seen the effects of cancer ripple through my life as I moved away from treatment, and I was insanely curious to know where I might be headed.

As I listened to our survivors' stories, I frequently—sometimes painfully—recognized where I had been. But, even better, I have been given tantalizing glimpses of where I might go. No excuses. No guarantees. Just the ability and strength to commit wholeheartedly to life. My life.

About Here and Now

IN THIS BOOK, we'll introduce you to thirty-nine very different people, all of whom have confronted cancer at some point in their lives. In their own words, they tell us who they are *today*, as a result of living through the disease.

The survivors on these pages are of all ages and come from all walks of life: a Texas rancher, a well-known feminist author, a housewife, a former gang member, and a pop star, just to name a few. They represent a wide range of diagnoses and treatments. Some were interviewed a few months out of treatment; some more than twenty years out.

Our hope is that there is someone in this book who reflects your own experience, whether you see yourself in his photograph or hear your thoughts echoed in her words. Whether you've had the disease or have survived some other trauma.

Cancer takes an enormous toll. Living beyond treatment presents particular demands. We witnessed how people moved on, incorporated, or ignored the disease. We were moved and, at times, affected by these stories. We listened and we learned—about others' experiences, about ourselves, about our invisible connections. The cancer experience is, in the end, uniting. It ties us to an extraordinary community of people—people who showed us that it is possible for any one of us, in the face of overwhelming adversity, to surprise ourselves with the depth of courage and strength that lies in us and those around us.

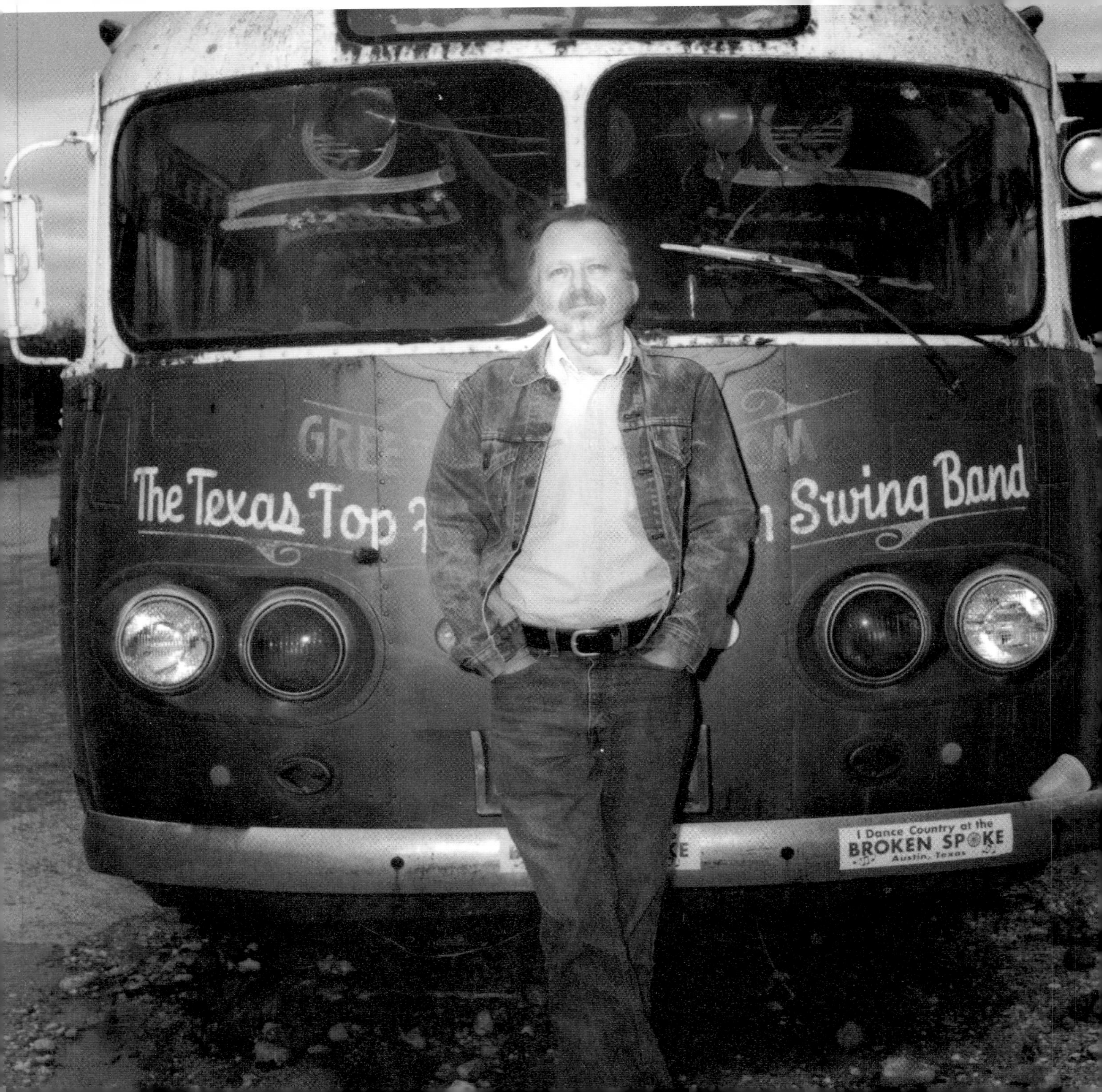
The Texas Top
Swing Band
I Dance Country at the
BROKEN SPOKE
Austin, Texas

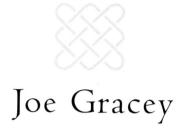

Joe Gracey

TWENTY-THREE-YEAR
SURVIVOR

SQUAMOUS CELL
CARCINOMA

I WAS DIAGNOSED when I was twenty-seven, which would have made it 1978. I was on the road doing radio promotions, driving from station to station. One day, I looked in the hotel mirror, wondering why my goddamn tongue just kept on hurting all the time. I pulled it out and saw a big ol' white circle the size of a dime on the underside of it and said "Jesus H. Fucking Christ!" It looked unnatural and alien, like it had landed on my tongue from outer space.

They decided that I should have radiation to the base of my tongue, which was where the cancer was. They hoped to reduce or kill the tumor cells and, with any luck, make surgery unnecessary and thus save my ability to speak. I was a singer and disk jockey, so I was looking at trying to save my livelihood at that point.

Today, I cannot speak. I use a child's Magic Slate to write to people, so extended answers to questions are a little bit harder than normal. On the slate I've learned to say everything I know in eight words or less, and long jokes are absolutely out of the question.

I didn't have to have chemo, although I had enough radiation to make my mouth permanently burned to this day. If I had to describe my cancer experience on my slate, it would read: "Terror. Repeated surgeries. Near-death experience. Better man."

I learned that life is very, very short, even if it is very long, and to get on it and ride it to the end of the line and not waste a moment of it, no more than you would waste a drop of cool water in the desert. I love harder and look closer and feel more.

I think at first I was trying to figure out why this happened to me at such a young age, so I looked at things like my smoking and drinking, both of which are considered to be contributing factors. But I figure that I wasn't doing anything that millions of twenty-seven-year-olds aren't doing. The fact that I developed cancer probably points to a genetic reason, either inherited from my great-grandfather—who also had an oral cancer—or a mutation, because I grew up downwind from a large U.S. nuclear testing site, and a disproportionate number of my classmates have had cancer.

I had the common misperception that cancer was some sort of evil, foreign thing that suddenly grows in you from nowhere. I was so terrified that I made the classic mistake of first ignoring the sore on my tongue, then going from doctor to doctor to try to avoid a biopsy until, finally, I had no choice. By then it was too late to save my tongue or larynx, or I would still be speaking today.

I've always been a rather ironic person, so that carried me through a lot of weird stuff, since I was able to just incorporate the weirdness into whatever I was doing and go on. The only way to deal with all of this is with a sense of humor, frankly. I mean, it continues to this day, because I have classic Frankenstein-looking scars and funny-looking pieces of tissue grafted into my neck, and people stare at me nonstop wherever I go. So I have to keep my sense of humor or I would just kill everybody at the grocery store.

I have learned that people stare because it is an involuntary human response to anything that is different. It is only our manners that cause us to look away, so I don't take it personally anymore, but I do think it is a pain in the butt, nonetheless. You got a choice: either get mad or laugh, and laughing is better. At one point I had a quarter-sized hole in the bottom of my mouth and had to tie a surgeon's mask with a bunch of cotton in it to catch the saliva as it dripped out of the hole. It looked like I was wearing a sanitary napkin under my chin. Try taking *that* to the grocery store sometime.

I was lucky enough to have great parents and two sets of wonderful grandparents, all of whom were good, strong people with toughness and love and a sense of humor. In a way, I had been prepared all my life for the cancer ordeal, since it is that combination of toughness and laughter that carried me through.

I was scared to death for five years. I went in all the time for checkups and biopsies, and I would sit out there in the waiting room for them to come out and tell me I was clean, or not. It was hell. I went about half-crazy; I should have been in mental-health counseling, but wasn't. After five years, I began to relax and deal with reality. Now, I am happy and no longer worry about cancer returning—it has been more than twenty years. I still miss my voice, naturally, especially the singing and the storytelling and joking around, since I was a good talker and it was a big part of who I am. But the mere lack of a speaking voice is a relatively insignificant thing compared to the glorious blessing of this life I lead.

I am a great listener. I also had to learn patience, because many things are frustrating or impossible for me now. It's a cliché, but the truth is that I really did begin to savor each moment of my life, even the tough stuff, because it is all good for something. I will literally never take one single second of my life for granted again, which is a great gift given to me by my cancer. I savor my family, my marriage, my kids, my wife—they all look like brilliant, shining jewels in my eyes. I savor my little convertible sports car, my dog, my house, and my body. The Buddha called it "mindfulness," and he was right about that— it is the best way to live. Perhaps I might have come to this place had I not had cancer, but it sure kicked me into high gear, so I have it to thank.

I learned that life is very, very short, even if it is very long, and to get on it and ride it to the end of the line and not waste a moment of it, no more than you would waste a drop of cool water in the desert. I love harder and look closer and feel more.

The human mechanism is tough, tougher than you realize until you have to pull the trigger on something as serious as the loss of your voice, or a leg, or a lung. I got to be sort of a pro at the whole hospital thing, which is in fact one way of coping with it—to get good at it. I was nice to the people who took care of me, because I appreciated what they did. I fell in love with all the nurses and told them so. I made my doctors understand that I appreciated what they knew, but that I was going to manage my own treatment as an equal with them.

I learned to be stoic, Zen, and to deal with the fear the same way I dealt with pain—encircle it, watch it, but don't participate in it completely. It is exactly like being the undersized linebacker on the high school football team: you see some big, giant running back coming straight at you, and you can either lie down on the ground and start crying, or you can stick your helmet in his sternum and lift him a foot off the ground as the light explodes inside your head from the impact. You get up, tell him he runs like your little sister, walk off the field, and throw up. Simple.

Today I am an engineer/producer, a bass player for my wife Kimmie's band, a copublisher, record-label mogul, Webmaster, Kimmie's manager, press-release writer, etc. We have our own little record label that we put her records on, and I help her with all of her career stuff. We are a sort of self-contained cottage industry. Sometimes I do outside projects too, like a Willie Nelson record or something fun like that. I'm a jack-of-all-trades, in other words.

I met Kimmie after I lost my voice, so she has never heard me utter a word. She claims that she is so used to the way I communicate with her, by signing and finger spelling, that she can't imagine it any other way. I am less likely to take everyday problems seriously. I am more forgiving, more patient. I guess I may have rubbed off on my family, because we have a pretty heavy commitment to celebration in our life. We celebrate every day, in fact, with good meals together at the table, or nights where we go out in the backyard and lay on a blanket together to look at the stars. We celebrate every possible birthday and Mother's Day and holiday to the hilt, no holds barred. Nothing goes untoasted or un-fêted around this house. That is how you mark the days, by celebrating them as they flash by. Otherwise, what do you have except nights in front of the TV or the computer or on the phone? Nights that you might as well have been dead, as far as I'm concerned.

I can't escape being a survivor, even if I wanted to. I'm proud of myself. I'm not foolish enough to think that I am special because I did that, only that I know something important now that maybe not everybody knows. I know that Death rides with me every moment of every day, but I do not fear him now, any more than I fear going to sleep at night. It is probably much like people who go off to war and find out that they are tough enough to fight and survive and lucky enough to come home.

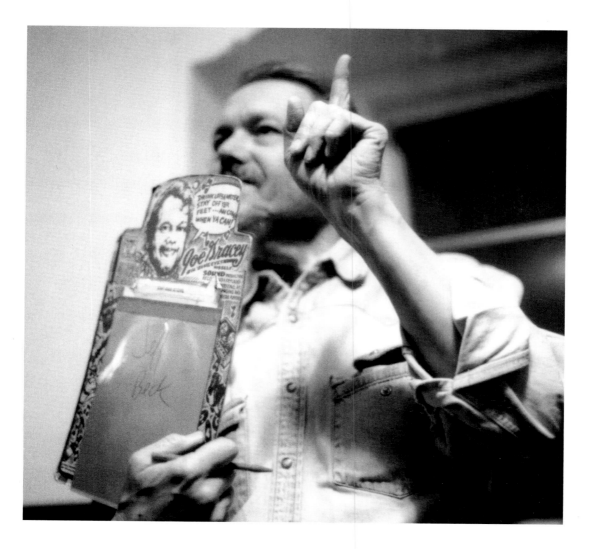

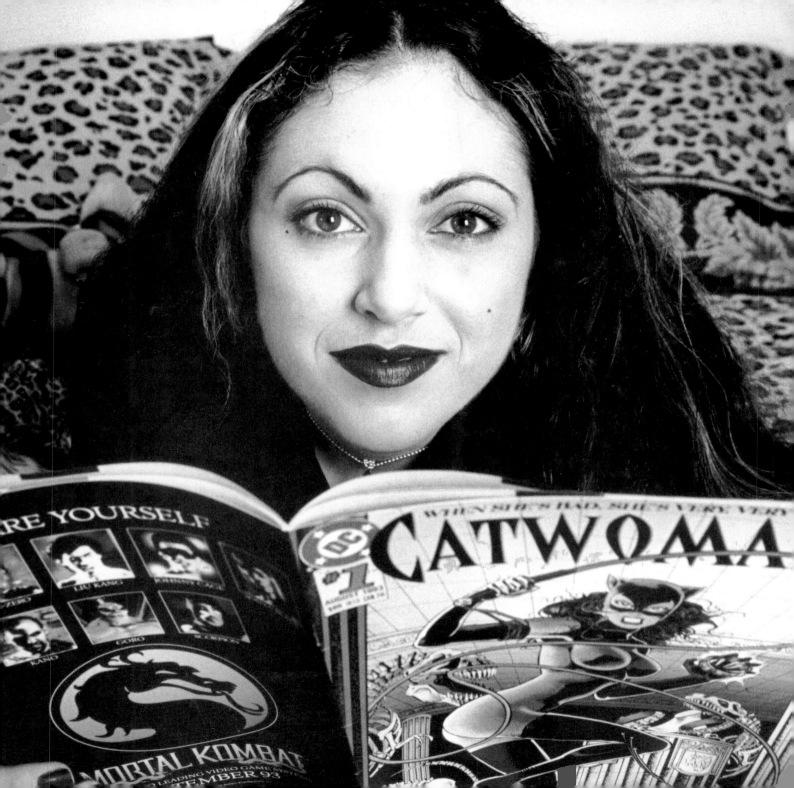

Margaret Gallagher

EIGHT-YEAR SURVIVOR
HODGKIN'S DISEASE

I'M TWENTY RIGHT now and live just outside San Francisco. I was diagnosed with Hodgkin's disease when I was a freshman in high school. My mother couldn't understand what was happening to me. I slept all the time. Doctors I saw said I was a typical teenager: moody and depressed; an only child. My mother bought me a dog to cheer me up.

I first found my tumor when I was in the shower and it finally clicked that something was really wrong with me. I had to go into the hospital and get an IV for a day, then I'd go home and take pills for two weeks after that. Then I'd do two weeks of radiation. I was on and off that routine for eleven months.

I didn't want to tell any of my friends about the cancer. I couldn't even go back to school. I didn't feel comfortable letting everyone see me as I was; as I'd become. So I stayed home and began hanging out with my two girlfriends in San Francisco a lot. I didn't want to be stopped from living my normal life. I wanted the long hair and the bangs and the eyeliner. And here I was, bald and wearing a wig.

I was angry. I wanted to be normal and I couldn't be. At fourteen you want to be like everyone else. My friends and I got in a lot of trouble together. We spray painted, snuck out of the house at night, shoplifted, and were really mean to our parents. Finally we got into so much trouble we weren't allowed to see each other anymore. By that time, I was relieved—I was tired of being bad. I wanted to go back to school, and when treatments stopped I did.

I was really scared. I wasn't scared about death but about what my body was going through, about the medicine and the way it made me feel. I think everyone was scared at that time. I know my parents were afraid they were going to lose their only daughter. My relationship with my mother is a whole lot stronger now. I think it's partly because of what we've been through together, and partly because I've grown up and matured. I was fourteen and supposed to hate my parents. But I needed them so much, too.

I'm the only one I know who gets full use out of my tiger print shoes.

About a year and a half after I was diagnosed, my parents found a group for teenagers with cancer in San Francisco. They made me go even though I was scared. I thought everyone would sit around the table talking about their feelings and that's the last thing I wanted. But no one talked about cancer; we just had fun. The Louis Group gave me the foundation to believe that I was still normal and could have friends who had cancer. I found people who had been diagnosed around the same time I was and we bonded. The boys thought I was cute, even though I wore a wig. I had great clothes and always had lipstick on.

Right now, I'm five years out of treatment and going to junior college. I also work at a beauty store in a mall—nothing exciting. My boyfriend is a big part of my life. He's twenty-six. He lost both his parents so he understands me. I gravitate toward people who understand anything about cancer. Then they can understand me.

When I was sick, I started going to a camp for kids with cancer. And it is still a very important part of my life. When I'm outside, spending time with the kids, I love life. I want to help other children know that they are normal, they just have cancer. At home, I walk around numb. But while I'm at camp, I can't do that because I feel so much more in touch with who I am. There I found my niche, and myself.

I know that if I didn't have cancer, I'd be a totally different person. I would barely have made it through high school. I'd probably have a kid. There would be nothing different about me. But I felt so different from others when I was going through treatments, it gave me the license to stay different. I'm confident now that if someone is going to like me, it's honestly because of who I am. I'm eccentric. I'm freer. I'm the only one I know who gets full use out of my tiger print shoes.

I am sad a lot now, but I don't feel guilty for surviving. I know that if I don't feel well emotionally, I won't feel well physically. I have peace with myself, although I do slip sometimes. I've lost a lot of friends, but I try to let things go and just live each day as it goes by. I reflect on death and how close I was to it—I could have reached out my arm to touch it. My priorities are in order now: friends and relationships come first.

Sometimes I still feel a lot of anger and want to do destructive things. That's why I totally relate to Catwoman. She's the coolest thing in the world. She sneaks out at night to steal jewelry for herself just because she loves it. She would never harm anyone or be mean. I want to have beautiful things, but I also want to do good.

My life does revolve around having cancer. But because of it, I've got more life to me. I believe that if I'm going to have something, I want it all. I can't just have one shade of vamp lipstick, I've got to have three. And also the lip liner, the brush, the palette, the blush. My experiences with cancer have made me want to enjoy life more, to really feel it, to wrap myself up in it. I want to roll around in life the way a dog rolls around in grass.

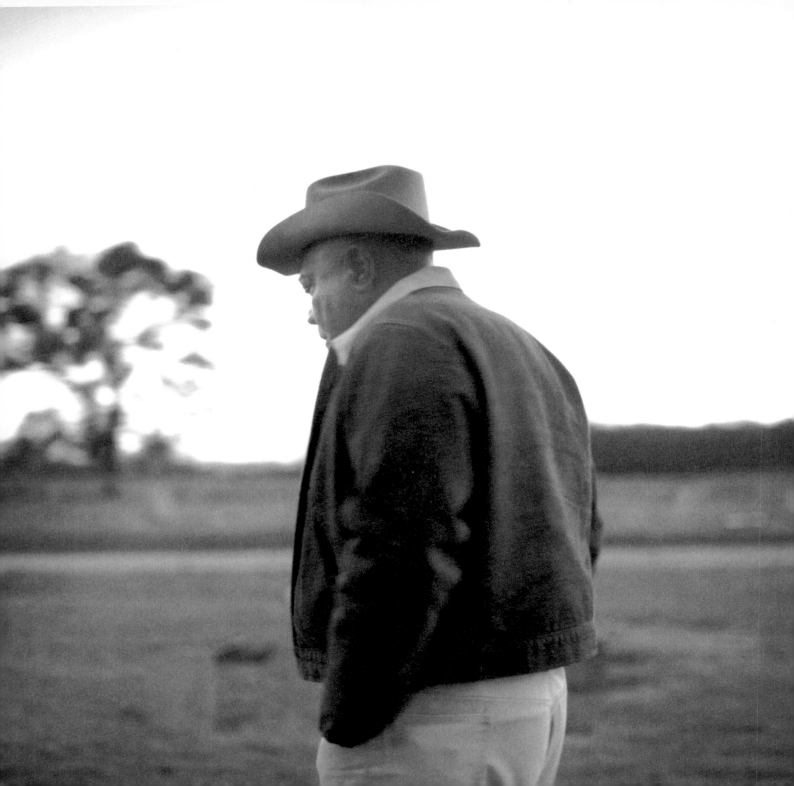

Bernard Porter

SEVEN-YEAR SURVIVOR

MALIGNANT FIBROUS
HISTIOCYTOMA

BACK WHEN I was about ten or twelve years old, I showed a calf in Corsicana, Texas. I won first place. The black boys, we had to be in a different pen and a different barn from the white boys. I was raised in an all-black community, and we had very little contact with whites. So the white boys and the agriculture teachers came over to look at the black boys' calves, and one white boy had a water gun and was shooting it at me. One of the richest men in Corsicana, a multimillionaire, was walking by with his wife and he said,

"Boy, if you don't get up and fight back you ain't never gonna be worth a damn." See, I was afraid. I thought if I hit him back they might put me in jail. So I had a walking stick, and I stood up and defended myself with it. What he said that day about fighting back always stuck with me. That's how I stood up against the cancer, too.

I had shipped a load of cattle in July or August of 1994. A little hard knot had formed on my leg about four or five inches above my knee. It was hard as a brick, but I thought a calf kicked me there. I didn't pay it no mind. It never did get sore, never did bother me or anything, so I went three or four months. My wife kept insisting, so I went down to my family doctor and he did a biopsy in December. It was malignant.

I had been doing farm work and ranch work all my life. Never been sick a day, other than a little back problem or whatever, but I hadn't really had a serious sickness. And it was a big shock to me when the doctor told me I had cancer. I couldn't sleep for two or three days or nights. When they said, "It's cancer," well, I thought I might live a few months and then that was gonna be it. It took me a good while to accept that a man living in the country, eating good food, in good health, not smoking, could get cancer. But I finally realized that we all can have anything, so then I accepted it. And with the help of my family and my doctor, I made it through all right.

I meet somebody and we get to talking, they say, "What you doing limping, Porter?" I say, "They had to cut part of my leg out. I had cancer." And he'll say, "Well, you know I had cancer," or "my mother had cancer," or "my father"—you know. Then I'll tell him about my experience and we'll talk. I always try to encourage them to get through it. Feels like I'm helping.

I owned several hundred head of cattle, but my doctor said to me, "Porter, if I was you, I'd forget about those cattle. I'd concentrate on myself." So I had to give up my cattle, but it wasn't that hard. I just forgot about outside interests. I prayed a lot and I concentrated my energy on myself and on getting well.

I was diagnosed with cancer just after my sixty-fifth birthday, when Medicare became available. I was thankful for that. I still have some of the bills. I guess I'm going to keep them as souvenirs, I don't know. Luckily my wife taught school and she had school insurance. Plus somebody had sold us a cancer policy, which paid off like a slot machine.

After I finished treatments, I couldn't get on a tractor too well. And I love horses, I've been a cowboy all my days, and I couldn't ride a horse. But I got a riding mower. I can mow the yard and get in my truck and ride over our land a little bit. Other than that, it curtailed a lot of my activity: riding around the pastures, checking fences. You have to adjust to certain conditions. So I did that. But it wasn't too difficult. I was sixty-six years old and I had worked hard all my days. I thought it was time for me to set up under the trees and watch the birds pass by, or do anything I wanted to do.

I love to go to town and carry my wife to the mall. I get me a chair and I set up and everybody who comes by, I meet 'em. I talk to 'em. I don't care what color they are, if she'll talk or he'll talk, I talk to 'em. We'll talk about the weather, talk about cattle, talk about whatever. Made some good friends that way.

When I go to the doctor's office, there's so many there I don't have a chance to talk to too many people. Most of them are in worse shape than I am. They're kind of depressed. But at the mall or town, I meet somebody and we get to talking, they say, "What you doing limping, Porter?" I say, "They had to cut part of my leg out. I had cancer." And he'll say, "Well, you know I had cancer," or "my mother had cancer," or "my father"—you know. Then I'll tell him about my experience and we'll talk. I always try to encourage them to get through it. Feels like I'm helping.

I get up every morning and I look at the morning dew and the sunshine and I thank the good Lord that I'm here to enjoy this day. I try to do something positive every day. I do work around the church, and I get some boys to help me cut the grass at the local cemetery every other week or so. And I'm on the board of a local nursing home, so I go down and give my two cents' worth. We make sure that the surroundings are good for the residents. That it don't smell bad, and that the folks in there get good care.

I want to see my grandkids all get grown and get fixed up in life or go through college or marry or whatever. I tell them that Grandaddy hopes he can help them. I have one little granddaughter, she says she's going to Texas A&M, and she wants me to buy her a new car when she goes. I told her to keep studying and work hard so she could get out of school and get a scholarship and finish college. And Jean and I will sure enough be there, with our walking canes and walkers.

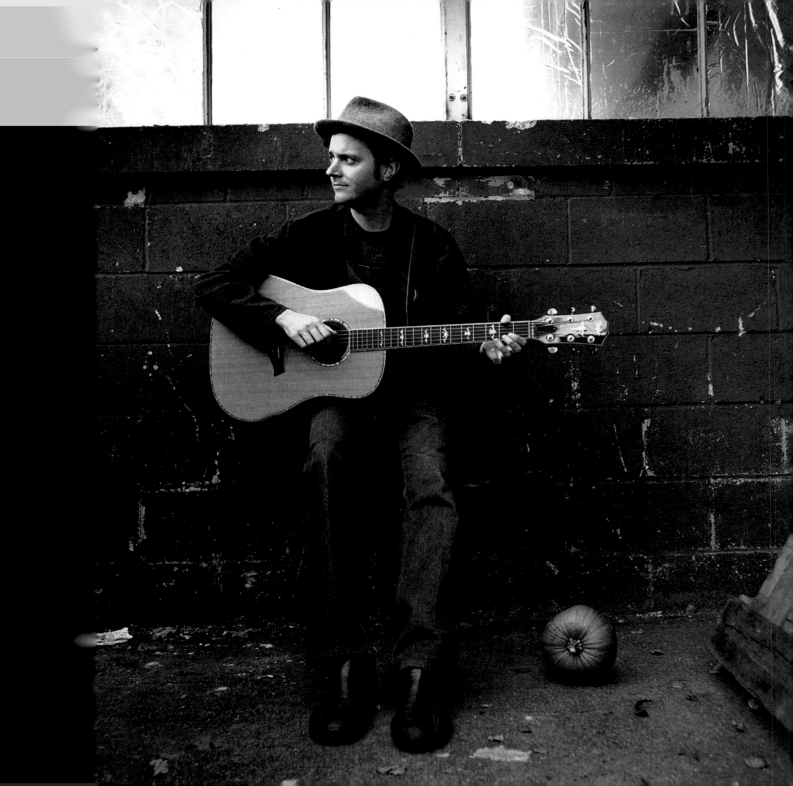

Kevin Hearn

TWO-YEAR SURVIVOR

LEUKEMIA

■

I HAD TWO things happen to me at once that many people don't have happen in a lifetime: I had cancer and a record
that went to number one on the charts. In the same week.
Now, I'm just trying to appreciate what's normal.

I'm in a band called the Barenaked Ladies. We were in a
studio making a record called *Stunt* at the time I was diagnosed. It was the first time I was recording with the band in
the studio, so I was very excited, very into it and wanted to
do a really good job, but I thought I was getting the flu or

something. We were all having a really good time, so the last thing I needed was to get cancer and ruin the whole thing. It was like a cruel joke. As if everything I'd worked for my whole life had been taken away from me; I wouldn't be able to enjoy it, and I might never get back to it. I'd worked really hard. My success was incentive to get well and get back to playing.

We were in *Rolling Stone* magazine and I had a copy of it beside my hospital bed. One day a nurse came in who didn't know me and she was looking through it. She said, "I don't know how these people do it, go on tours and play in shows." And I wanted to say, "Look at that picture—that's me!" My identity had been taken from me.

I feel old now, post-cancer and post–bone marrow transplant. I feel more weary and wise. It all just seems like such a long time ago, before I was diagnosed, but I think about it every day. It comes up in different forms; my experience was pretty public, so whoever I run into— someone I know or don't know—they usually ask me how I'm doing. I know it's more than a "How are you doing?" It's like an, "Am-I-going-to-see-you-again how are you doing?"

I had a lot of family support, especially from my sister, Mary Pat. She was there whenever I needed something. She was also there when I needed to do something I didn't want to do, like check into the hospital. One night I was sitting out on the porch with a cup of tea and a candle and she came down and said, "I really think you should go to the hospital, you're not doing so good." And I got mad at her. I didn't want to go. She went upstairs—at which point I managed to spill hot tea on my leg and light my pants on fire. I went upstairs and said to her, "I think you're right. Let's go."

Because my diagnosis was so public, I received an unbelievable amount of support: emails, letters, phone calls from fans and musicians. Musicians I respect and am not even close to were phoning me up. At first the band and I didn't know what to do about the diagnosis—to keep it private or make it known. But then we knew it wasn't something to be ashamed of. The experience was negative in the sense that it kind of became my identity; I stopped thinking of myself as a musician or an artist, and started thinking of myself as a cancer patient. But that's fading away now.

I don't think I can separate the experience from who I am, because it influences everything I do. I actually tap into it for inspiration in terms of writing music, or making decisions. That's the serendipity of it, I suppose.

When I was sick, I continued to play. I took my guitar into the hospital and wrote music. The medication I was on made me so shaky that at times I couldn't play. But as I got my strength back, I knew I didn't want to just sit at home for the year it was going to take me to get through it all. I used to go for walks. At first I could make it half a block. One day I received an email from Lou Reed, who's been a hero of mine for years. He had made a record called *Magic and Loss* about the cancer experience of two friends of his, which really helped me. That got back to Lou, and he wrote me an email saying, "I just wanted to tell you I was thinking of you and hope you're getting well and getting back to your music soon." That day, I walked all the way around the block.

One day, while I was walking, I ran into an old friend of mine who plays the bass. I told him about a few songs I'd been working on and he started coming over to my place every day. Eventually we went into the studio. I'd take a taxi over and sometimes I'd just lie on the couch and try and do as much as I could, or sit in the chair and play guitar. I really love the record we made. The songs are about transcending desperate situations. I think it helped me to get better.

For the few months that I couldn't play because I was too shaky, I realized what a gift it was to be able to play. I knew music wasn't something to be taken for granted; that it was a responsibility. That changed my attitude about how I lived my life and what I did musically. I felt so helpless without music. I've learned to dig deeper. I've learned the healing powers of music and I want to keep exploring that with future records.

I think I come across as kind of quiet and indecisive. But I knew I could get through this. I also had a weird feeling that I was going to go through a test like this in my life. So when it happened, in a weird way I wasn't surprised. I was ready for it. I had thought of my mortality before cancer, but in a strange way, romanticizing death. I thought about what music would be played at my funeral—"Walk on the Wild Side," or something like that.

When the band went back on the road to tour, we were all in a bit of denial. Eventually, I had to leave again because I almost bit the big one. I got sick on the road with graft vs. host disease—a whacking bad case of it. It's basically the new immune system rejecting the marrow. They gave

I don't think I can separate the experience from who I am, because it influences everything I do. I actually tap into it for inspiration in terms of writing music, or making decisions. That's the serendipity of it, I suppose.

me lots of drugs to help my body function and to suppress my immune system. I was on prednisone, which made me really puffy. My cousin called me Pumpkin Head. That was the hardest part. Prednisone fucks up your thinking. I was trying to explain it to my band mates: you can see your personality and you know it's there and you know who you are, but you can't access it. It's behind glass. The prednisone is running the show and you're an absolute asshole. Needless to say, that was a drag. I was on such high doses that it threw off my blood sugar levels and I became diabetic, which also screws up your thinking. I was just a mess.

I felt alienated from everyone. I wasn't me. My head was huge and I'd walk by people I knew on the street and they wouldn't recognize me, but I didn't have the heart to tell them. I felt like a ghost. I started feeling less like that about a year ago, when I finally got off that stuff.

Getting back on stage was tough. I performed when I was on prednisone. I don't remember a thing about it. I was told we played some of our best shows but I don't know how I even knew what parts to play. I felt incredibly self-conscious. No one could have comprehended how I was feeling, or why I was so set on working. I was just working to fight for my identity, to fight for my life.

I have a new identity now and I'm trying to embrace it. I'm not fighting for who I was but who I can be. I wanted a new everything, but I'm still figuring it all out. I'm still letting it go and putting it behind me. There are moments when I'm achieving something now and I feel like it's a marker, but the last year has been trying to just feel better and get my energy back. And be able to work again and have lunch with friends or see a band play—stuff I couldn't do for a long time that I appreciate now.

I still have a bit of fatigue. I used to be energetic—I could just go, go, go. I find my concentration and my focus and my memory were all affected, but I'm looking forward to those things coming back. All those drugs have side effects. They did a number on my bones. I was asked to play hockey last week and I thought, "If I fall on the ice, I'm going to shatter like a frozen piece of licorice." I think about those things now.

I want to be able to help people who might be going through this, to help give them courage and understanding of what it's like. I'd like to keep doing things to promote awareness of cancer and encourage people to support research and a healthier lifestyle. (Although I'm not one to talk—I just ordered a pizza.) The band has done concerts and donated ticket sales to the hospital where I was treated. We've played for patients and staff. We also invited the Cancer

Society of Canada to set up booths at our shows. We want to help register potential marrow donors. I always wanted to use my talent and visibility to raise money for good things.

I sometimes think about recurrence and I get a sinking feeling. But it's not happening today, so I'm just going to enjoy. Sometimes I think I work so hard because I'm trying to get so much done before anything happens to me. I worry that it's a bad thing to do. But as long as I'm enjoying it, I guess it's okay.

I think a lot about time. On my own record I talk about time and my relationship to it: "Only time will tell if there's a heaven or a hell, but time is weird, it has a beard and I don't know if I even want to know."

In my music, I'm trying to find new things to draw on. It all seems so light in comparison. I do and I don't like the intensity cancer brought to my life. I know my record has helped people because I've heard from them. And Lou Reed said it was a beautiful record. He told me that it is very important. That I've been somewhere most people don't go, and I have come back to report on it.

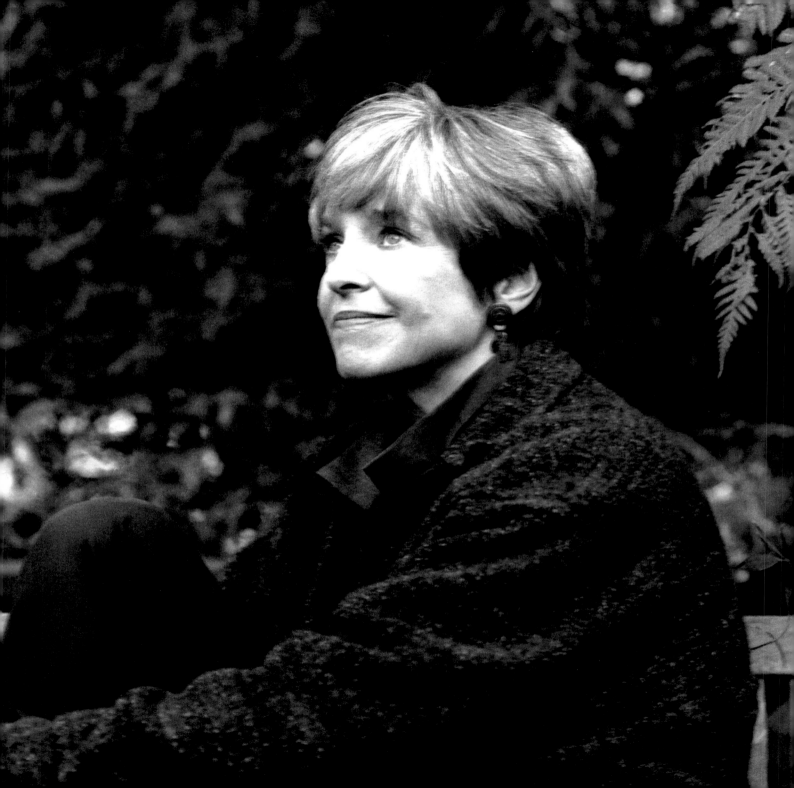

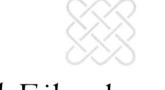

Jill Eikenberry

FIFTEEN-YEAR SURVIVOR
BREAST CANCER
■

I WAS DIAGNOSED IN 1986. Michael and I were in New York, but we'd come to Los Angeles to make the pilot for *L.A. Law* and we were going to be moving there for our big debut. We had two months between the pilot and the next episode, and that's when I found out I had breast cancer.

I found the lump when I checked myself while I was driving to a routine exam. I wasn't used to doing that, but I had been scheduled for my first mammogram by my doctor and I think I might have subconsciously checked myself. And I've often thought there was something intuitive about it, because women tend to have this ability. I was very frightened because I'd never felt anything like that before.

I tried to be as optimistic as possible. People I'd talked to said not to worry; it was just a benign cyst, everyone has them. I had more pictures and went to see a breast specialist. Michael and I were both still hoping that it was benign, but we knew from the pictures that it wasn't. That was another moment of truth, when the doctor said it was malignant.

I thought I was going to die. The doctor suggested either a lumpectomy or a mastectomy, with mastectomy being his choice because that's what he did most often. I said, "Do whatever you have to do to get it off of me." We went home and I really felt that my life was over. I was in total despair.

I had the love of my husband to comfort me, but I was pretty numb for the first few days. I called a friend who gave me a doctor's name for a second opinion. He was much less conservative and he became my surgeon. He said I didn't need to lose my breast. The big thrust for me over the last ten years has been networking to find other women with the same diagnosis and similar treatment, so that they can see that it's not the end of the world. But at that point I didn't have anyone with whom to network. People weren't talking about breast cancer.

At the time, I had a four-year-old son and a sixteen-year-old daughter, and I did everything wrong in terms of communication. The sixteen-year-old was hard to communicate with in the best of times and it was really hard to tell what she was thinking. She was my husband's daughter from his first marriage, but I'd raised her from a baby and she was feeling a lot of things she's only recently told me. We did a wonderful workshop together where she said that she had been afraid to hug me because she thought she would hurt me or that I would break. We didn't tell our son anything because we thought he was too young to be able to deal with it. But soon after I got home from the hospital he came to me and asked, "Mom, are you going to die?" So that was clearly not the right way to go with him, because he had all kinds of frightening scenarios in his mind.

We called the producer in L.A. and said that I had cancer and we couldn't do the show. He said that I should come, that he would figure out a way for me to do my radiation at UCLA after work. When he said, "Jill's not going to die this way," we thought he was God and, of course, we believed him. I had my lumpectomy in New York, and they took out eleven nodes, all of which were negative. The operation was a success; I was in good shape. Then we flew to L.A., where I had my radiation.

We were very frightened and told only our very closest friends. Nobody in the cast knew the situation. I felt there was such a stigma attached to it. I didn't want to be known as the woman with cancer instead of this new, vibrant attorney, Ann Kelsey. I felt ashamed. It wasn't until a few years later, when I was approached by a woman who is a documentary filmmaker and producer who also had breast cancer, that I began to talk to other women about it. Almost universally, they talked about what an amazing thing it is to have this disease and get through it and come out the other side. And most of the women had felt ashamed about having breast cancer.

What was amazing for me was that my aunt Treeva, my mother's oldest sister who'd had it forty-five years before, had a double radical mastectomy and had been burned badly from the radiation, then gotten right back on her tractor in Ohio. I never knew about it. I didn't know she didn't have any breasts!

For me, it seemed as if it would affect my career adversely if I came out with it. Once I did come out, it was just the opposite. I became much more in demand after that. Not just for acting, but for speaking situations and addressing women. I went through a period when I thought, "Okay, enough of breast cancer. I want to get on with it. I'm done with it." But in the last few years Michael and I decided to go on the speaking circuit. A lot of what we have to say has to do with our relationship. Because of the cancer, we made a huge shift in our life. We'd always had a good relationship, but it then became *the* priority around which everything else revolved.

We do our breast cancer talk all around the country to audiences that are usually 50 percent breast cancer survivors. The breast cancer was a catalyst for our lives to become so much better. This is a message we like to share with breast cancer survivors because they are actually

We are our own worst enemies in terms of our fulfillment. So many of the women I've talked to who have survived breast cancer—or are in the throes of it—say that they have never even considered the idea of putting themselves first. I think I've learned to put myself first on my priority list and that we, as a couple, have learned to put our relationship first.

examining what their lives might be about. A lot of people don't want to look, but breast cancer survivors do.

Before I got sick I put much more emphasis on success. It's ironic that I got my mortality call and my immortality call at the same time. I think that the combination of the breast cancer and the success that I'd always wanted was great, because if I'd never been able to grab the brass ring I might never have been able to see the other side.

I just realized that my focusing on fulfillment, by being more honest about what I want and not lying about it—not telling half-truths or pretending, or saying I want something when I don't—has made me much happier on a day-to-day basis. Because I don't have any resentment toward my husband or children or anybody, they can flower. It's as if I'm fountaining over into them, as opposed to giving to them from a place of scarcity or emptiness, which is where women are so often coming from.

We are our own worst enemies in terms of our fulfillment. So many of the women I've talked to who have survived breast cancer—or are in the throes of it—say that they have never even considered the idea of putting themselves first. I think I've learned to put myself first on my priority list and that we, as a couple, have learned to put our relationship first.

Now people are talking about sexuality at breast cancer conferences. A lot of women who have had breast cancer feel that their lives are over in that department, but it's quite the opposite. I'm fifty-one, have been menopausal for five or six years and have no estrogen to speak of. But now I have more of a life force—libido—than I've ever had. There is just no need to stop being turned on because of hysterectomy, biopsy, or mastectomy. Our bodies are amazing, but we just don't give them any credit.

At this point, I feel more well than I have ever in my life, even long before my cancer. I don't think of myself as a person with a disease. I don't fear recurrence except when I go for my mammogram and sit in that booth waiting for the results. It's interesting that I spend so much time with people with cancer, yet it doesn't have me waking up in the middle of the night. It took a long time for that, but by the time I passed the five-year mark I stopped thinking about it every day.

I think the main thing that came out of the breast cancer scare was an acknowledgment that we're all going to die. Maybe I wasn't quite paying attention to that before and that's where my drive came from—my inability to "get" how much I have, and always having to go for something I didn't have. Rather than think about, "What if I die tomorrow?" I'd rather live today.

I've become more spiritual and I like feeling that I'm part of something much bigger. I meditate every day. I used to have a lot of nighttime fear of death and I don't anymore. I've lost a lot of that fear with meditation and the unbelievably profound connection I've developed with my husband.

I truly believe that we all want intimacy and connection. I think that breast cancer has helped me with that. I could be made very afraid by the woman who tells me her stem cell transplant didn't work and she's got three months to live. That's what we're all afraid of. But if you keep looking into her eyes and hugging her, knowing that she's going to die and you are going to die, death loses its power.

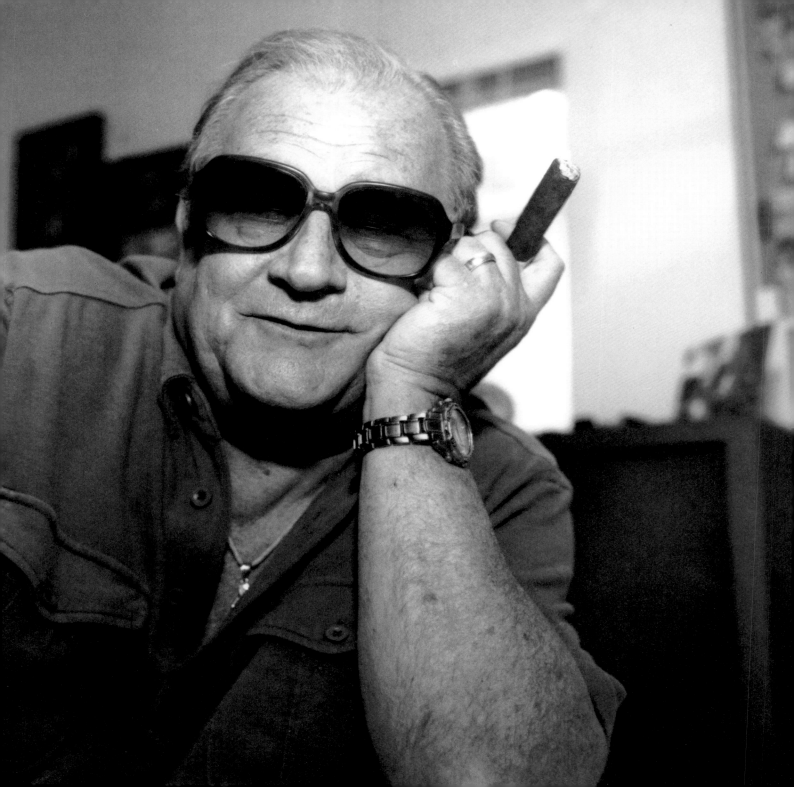

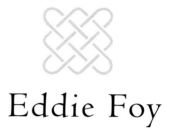

Eddie Foy

TWENTY-EIGHT-YEAR
SURVIVOR

MELANOMA, BLADDER
CANCER

*I*N 1973, I had a big, black mole on my leg that had split wide open. The doctor told me I had a very bad melanoma, and that it had to come off immediately. I said, "I don't have time for surgery." I was casting seven shows for Warner Brothers. I said, "Let's do this in March," and he told me, "You'll be dead in March." I said, "What are you doing tomorrow morning?"

I've gotten cancer twice—the second time it was bladder cancer, in April of 1995. I was in the middle of doing the

Jerry Lewis telethon when I was diagnosed. They took it out, put a catheter in me at nine o'clock, and took me back to work an hour and a half after the operation. I've had no recurrence since then.

Cancer turned out to be the best thing that ever happened to me. First of all, I quit drinking. I was obviously very unhappy in my home life, because I weighed 240 pounds when I got on the table. I was an ultra, ultra, ultra-right-wing conservative who believed that anyone with long hair had to be gay as a thirty-five-dollar bill. My whole life was confined to blinders. I didn't like me.

Cancer changed my life because I can never again be afraid of the truth. I know there's something stronger than me. I don't know if there's a heaven and a hell—I haven't been there. And I'm not about to go yet.

After my first surgery, I started to realize there were things out there like clouds, and sun. I started to realize that different people had ideas that I wanted to hear. There was music I wanted to listen to. I wanted to really get back to nature, which I had never done because I'm a New York City kid. And I made the momentous decision to leave my marriage.

Before cancer, I didn't think anything in the world could knock me down. I was a boxer—my nickname was the Bear. I was a very angry man as I grew up; I would fight at the drop of a hat. I never thought anything could hurt me, so when I saw this mole, I thought, "Oh, that's nothing." And I'd scratch it and pick it and not pay any attention. I'm a schmuck—what else can I say?

When I didn't like something, I ran away. Turned my back on it and just walked out of the room. Screw it. But this, I said to myself, I gotta take this mother head-on. 'Cause this is *bad*. This is not somebody hitting you with a right hand, this isn't losing a job—this was BAD. There was a chance that I wasn't going to be around to watch my daughter graduate from high school. She was the one who gave me all of the impetus to live.

The minute my eyes open in the morning now, I look up and I say inside my heart, "Thank you for giving me another day." Then I kiss my wife and get out of bed. But there isn't a day that goes by that I don't think about cancer, and I don't ever want that fear to go away. Because it's a positive fear, not a negative fear. I check everything every day. I make sure my wife, Jan, examines herself all the time. Feel your lymph nodes at least once a week. You've gotta dig down there. It may hurt, but you've got to stick your hand in your groin and see if there's anything swollen underneath there.

Anybody that doesn't is crazy. I know so many people—myself being one—who didn't pay attention to things like a mole that changed color or a lump in their breast. My philosophy is: GET THY ASS IN TO SEE YOUR DOCTOR NOW. Don't wait six months.

I do this, but at the same time, I don't sit around in a dark room with a freakin' cinnamon candle and say, "Oh, God, where are you gonna give it to me again?" I don't have time for that shit. I really don't. It may come back. Okay, let's take care of it. Move on. You want to lick this sucker, you can. But it can beat you. It's like Joe Louis: when he was ready to throw the right hand and your chin was there, forget it. You were knocked out. But for thirteen rounds, fight it.

I think fear can be such an overwhelming black shadow, that people forget they are more powerful than any fear that can be thrown at them. When people hear the word *cancer*, they hear D-E-A-T-H—it's like a panic comes over them. They don't think about all the options that are out there now. I mean, you educate yourself and move on. Now I think I'm more afraid of having a stroke or a heart attack.

I was a very powerful, physical man at one time. I'm careful now. I love my bourbon, I love a good cigar, I love my kids, but I watch myself. The doctor finally told me, no more sun. I used to put on a batch of crap that I made and lie in the sun all day; now, as long as the sun's out there, it's fine for me. No big loss. If I ain't gonna be around to see my daughter or my wife, smoke my cigars, listen to Rodgers and Hammerstein, or see the next future heavyweight champion of the world—that's the big loss.

Cancer changed my life because I can never again be afraid of the truth. I know there's something stronger than me. I don't know if there's a heaven and a hell—I haven't been there. And I'm not about to go yet.

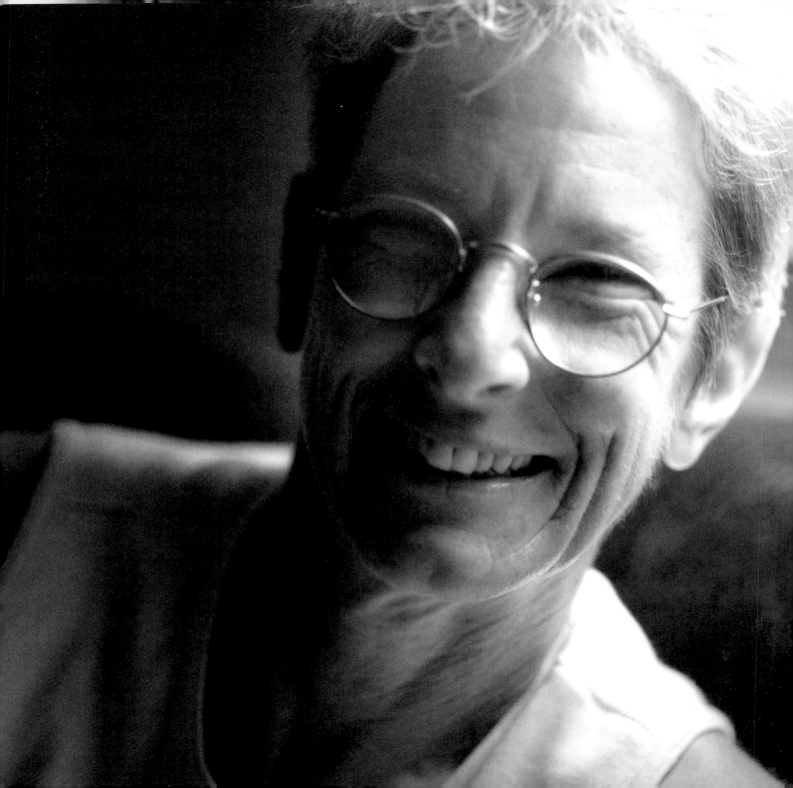

Karen Cole

THREE-YEAR SURVIVOR
ANAL CANCER

I WAS BICYCLING maybe five or six thousand miles a year, riding at least sixty or seventy miles a week. I went to a routine doctor's visit and he said I had hemorrhoids. So I just ignored it and went on cycling. Finally the thing just got enormous and it started to interfere with my seat, and when the doctor looked at it again, he said, "I think it's something else." They did a biopsy and it came back squamous-cell, HPV-related anal cancer.

Everything changed. I went from riding, literally the weekend before, in a one hundred-mile event, to being really ill—not from the cancer, but from the treatment. I had third-degree burns from my belly button all the way through my vaginal area up to my spine. I lost over 30 percent of my body weight.

I had related totally with my body because everything was performance-driven. I knew what to feed it, what to give it, what not to give it, when I was doing an event right and performing well. And what I lost from the treatment was my body. I didn't know who I was anymore. I couldn't work and I couldn't ride my bicycle and I couldn't depend on my body, which I had trusted. Where does your trust come from when there's no foundation?

In accepting death, it's like I'm finally living. And living is really important to me. It's living in the moment and not thinking about what my future might look like. I go bike riding every weekend. It's certainly crossed my mind that I might do other things, but what I really like is just living an ordinary life: going to work, getting up in the morning, going cycling—just living, you know?

As soon as the company I was working for found out I had cancer— I was V.P. of marketing—they fired me immediately. I was badly in debt from medical bills. I had no job, no money, and my car was repossessed. I was living with another woman at the time, my lover, and she had taken up the support for me 100 percent. On top of that, I became addicted to the morphine I was taking for the pain of my burns. I had gone from being healthy and self-sufficient and employed to being extremely dependent, drug-addicted, and burned. I wasn't capable of taking care of myself at all. Finally, I was admitted to drug rehab but, by that time, my relationship with my lover was destroyed as well.

She literally put me out on the street. Everything I identified with as being who I was, was now gone, and I was terrified. Coming out of the first round of cancer was, in a lot of ways, more terrifying than having cancer.

Before, I was always very self-sufficient. And one of the things I learned along this path was to accept help. I never asked my friends for anything, but one friend said I could live with her and I didn't have to pay rent. Another friend bought me a car, because my credit rating was so bad. I started looking for another job with an executive recruiter. Now I'm director of audience development for a dotcom company.

Going back to work, during the interview process, cancer was never mentioned. I was proud of myself for having survived, but at the same time I couldn't bring it up. You want to say, "Look! I just went through all this and yet, here I am, sitting here in front of you, and capable of coming to work." On the other hand, you really can't say that, because if they knew how horrible it was, they couldn't handle it.

I was rediagnosed a year after I finished treatment. I started chemotherapy again, but because of the last treatment, my bone marrow was so suppressed that it made me really sick right away. I was immediately unable to work. The thing is, my cancer is incurable. They can maybe prolong my life a teeny bit, but the chemo wouldn't kill the cancer, and the quality of my life would nosedive. So I decided not to do it. Just to live, and let the cancer go. And also, at the same time, plan what my death would be.

I'm fine with the fact that I'm dying. In accepting death, it's like I'm finally living. And living is really important to me. It's living in the moment and not thinking about what my future might look like. I go bike riding every weekend. It's certainly crossed my mind that I might do other things, but what I really like is just living an ordinary life: going to work, getting up in the morning, going cycling—just *living*, you know?

This society thinks about death as being a linear thing. You're born, and then you live as long as you can stay alive. And as soon as you start getting old—or old-looking—you do everything in your power to make yourself stay young-looking. But in other cultures, life and death are a continuous circle. And death is always there with you. At any moment, anybody could die. And if you know death is right there with you, wouldn't you live your life differently?

After the second diagnosis, I went back to the company and I told them. I got overwhelming support. Since that time I've been promoted; I'm now on the executive committee for the company. My discussion of my cancer and my health inside this company is open and it's out. Everyone knows what my prognosis is; everyone knows what it was like for me to go through treatment and to have to make the decision not to do treatment again.

I had to bring my friends and family around. I've had to literally drag some of them kicking and screaming up to this point. My daughter had one big cry. Since then, we've discussed all of these things and she knows exactly what I want, and she's fine with that. She still says, "Oh,

Mom. You won't be here to see my children." But I can't go there. I cannot think about that. Because that gets into causing myself emotional pain.

I've been reading a lot of books along the Buddhist line that talk about the difference between pain and suffering. For instance, you drop a hammer on your foot. That causes pain. But that's not suffering. Suffering comes into it when you attach an emotional reaction to it. When you say, "Damn you for leaving that hammer out!" Now you're suffering, because now you're blaming someone else.

I could suffer from my cancer, I could say, "Oh, God . . . woe is me . . . I have cancer. I feel so bad. Ooohh, I'm gonna die!" And I could create this whole world of suffering and pity; I could get myself into a real funk about the whole thing. Or I could go the other way and say, "Okay, I have cancer. I accept it." And when I have pain, acknowledge that it's there, but don't turn it into suffering by saying, "Oh, my cancer's growing, it's spreading!"

One of the things the doctor asked me was whether I wanted ongoing tests, and I said no. I don't want updates on where it's metastasized to the next minute, you know? As I feel it,

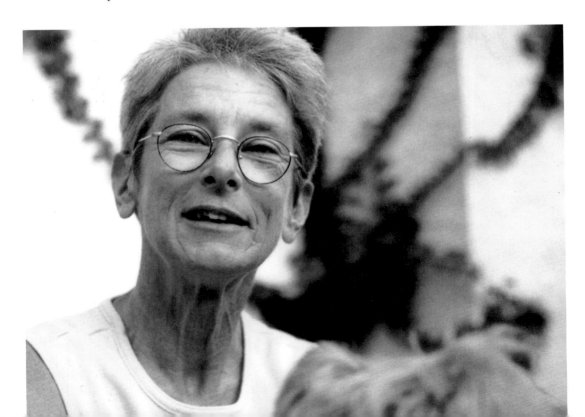

then we'll deal with it. So when the pain does come, it won't be pain from suffering; it'll be, "Oh, gee. I have a pain in my right groin over there. Isn't that interesting? Oh, the quality of that pain is, it's intense," or, "It's kind of dull." And that's how I acknowledge it.

In the horror and terror of my first round of treatment, something clicked inside of me. Now I am able to dissociate from it quite a lot, because I understand absolutely that this has nothing to do with me. And I think that was the biggest hurdle of overcoming it, realizing that cancer's not attacking the essence of who I am, it's attacking my body. My body is basically a vessel that holds who I am in it, and who I *am* has really nothing to do with my physical body.

Honestly, cancer has been the best thing. It has abruptly brought me to awareness and made me really active in choosing my path and life. Who would have known that cancer could come in and at first seem like the most destructive force that ever hit, and then turn out to be the most positive thing that ever happened? It really has been a gift and continues to be; I wouldn't be where I am today, or feeling like I do feel today, if it hadn't been for cancer. I certainly do not ever see myself as a victim, ever. I am a survivor and I'm really proud of that.

The essence of your life is the relationships that you have. What I think comes after, what I truly believe, is that I go on. Not as Karen Cole, but the fundamental essence of who I am—whatever that is—goes on. I'm not afraid. I'm not hoping for a miracle. It's not like I'm looking at clinical trials all the time thinking, "Oh, at any moment they're going to be able to save Karen Cole!" It's okay. There's a quote from Sitting Bull when he's going to be executed. He says, "Today is a good day to die, because all the things of my life are present in this moment." That's how I feel. And *that's* what brings the comfort and the peace.

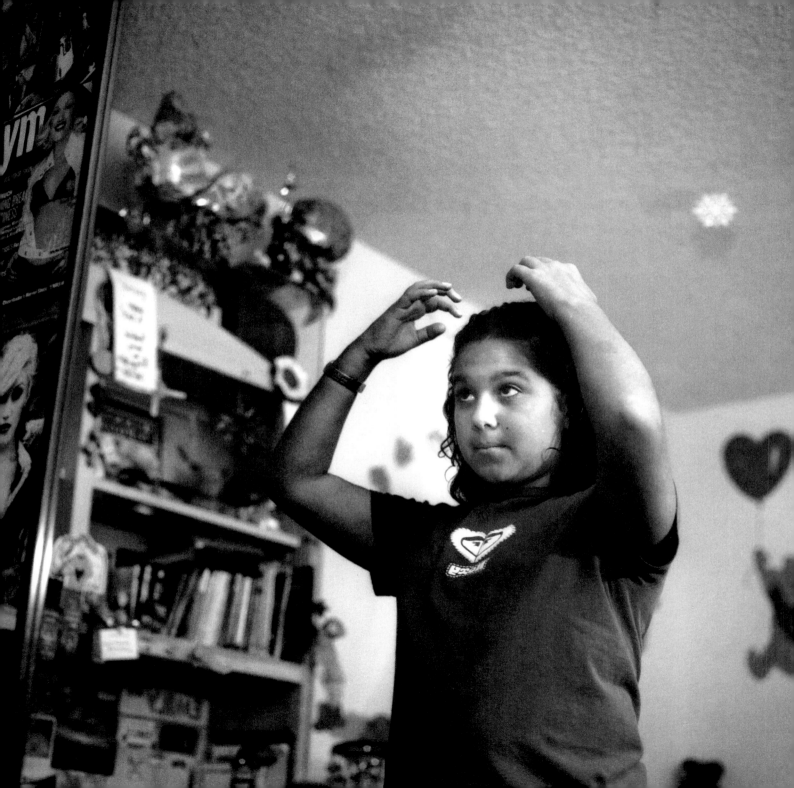

Emily Olvera

PARENTS: *Patty and Bob Olvera*

FOUR-YEAR SURVIVOR
LEUKEMIA

■

I AM TWELVE years old and I was diagnosed at the beginning of 1997 with leukemia, with the Philadelphia chromosome. It was really rare, so it was very, very scary for our family.

I had just turned seven. I remember the very first day perfectly. The doctor came in and all of a sudden I saw everyone break out in tears. My parents explained to me that I had a sickness and what the risks were. I had no idea what they were talking about, but I remember crying when I heard that I was going to lose my hair.

I have two older sisters. My thirteen-year-old sister I didn't get to see at all because she was at school every day, but me and my twenty-three-year-old sister got really close. She would spend the night with me in the hospital and do everything with me. My dad and mom suspected that my middle sister would be a little bit jealous because I got a lot of gifts, money, and cards, but actually she wasn't. It brought our whole family closer together.

In a way, I think cancer pushed me to grow up faster than I needed to, but I'm trying to be who I am, and I'm a kid.

PATTY AND BOB: *Our twenty-three-year-old daughter was very involved with Emily's treatment, but our thirteen-year-old was very much in denial. She didn't want to talk about it, hear about it. She actually regressed a little bit; started refusing going into dark places of the house by herself. We recognized that and tried to help. I'm sure there were times when we overcompensated with our middle daughter; I'm sure there were times we undercompensated as well.*

I got homeschooled for second and third grade. All I thought about was my friends and I was so sad not being able to see them. They couldn't come over because I couldn't have any contact with other people; basically only doctors, nurses, and my family. I felt like I was being left out.

I know my body better now because I know what's going on in it. I never used to think about it, but now I do; about the platelets, the blood cells, and everything like that because when I had my chest tube in, I would always do my own cleanings.

There have been some people in the hospital who passed away. I noticed that it's almost always the ones who never felt high, who never thought about the good things in life. Their rooms were dark. I always found something to do in the hospital, like make beads or bracelets—all different kinds of things.

BOB: *We talked about death and dying with our family. Emily asked me because I was a doctor, if I would know if she was going to die. When I told her yes, she said, "Will you tell me?" And I told her I would, so it wasn't something to be afraid of. These kids know anyway. Without our telling them, these kids know.*

They're smarter than we think they are, they're more aware than we think they are and I think it only helps if you can address the issues and talk with them about it.

I got closer to my parents. We spent time at home together and talked about things. That was a good feeling, but I knew that I was taking my parents away from other people, and that was not a good feeling. I appreciated so much that they were caring for me and loving me during that time.

To me, cancer meant many hardships, pain, suffering, and loss of friendship. A lot of people say I shouldn't have to go through that when I'm just a kid. I feel that I can do almost anything now if I could survive two years of chemotherapy.

PATTY: *Some of the kids were jealous of Emily. We didn't expect that. We had to explain to her teachers what was going on, so they were all aware of what she went through and sometimes they favored her a little bit. Also, we sought out a lot of public support, so the Anaheim Angels and the Mighty Ducks did some things for her. She got to meet Celine Dion. She'd tell the kids and even some of her best friends would say, "You're bragging." She said to them, "You know what? I'll trade with you. You want to have the cancer? I'll give you all the stuff I got."*

I was so nervous the night before going back to school. What if my friends weren't going to hang around me? What if people stared? And they did stare, so much. A lot of people at school did make fun of me, but I talked to them about it and I said, "You know what, it's not cool that you're doing this," and they stopped. A lot of my friends stood up for me, too.

I was a little shy about my appearance because either I had gained weight or I was super, super skinny. But somebody should never judge you on that. It doesn't matter what's on the outside, it just matters who I am and what I'm living for.

I don't make fun of people, but sometimes I go along with my friends. But if it gets out of hand and they're being very mean, I say, "Don't do that." They can't get to know a person if they're going to make judgments about him or her.

Some days I want to be an adult and do those things my parents won't let me. But then I want to stay a kid, because I've already learned a lot of things that maybe an adult wouldn't even know.

Cancer is still in my everyday life, but I don't think about it as much as I did. If I see a bruise on my arm, I think, "Oh my gosh, am I getting it again?" When I went on maintenance I was very scared it would come back. I think about it at the oddest times, like when I'm having fun at the mall.

My family just got back from Hawaii two weeks ago. I'm so happy we went because I look at life when I'm on vacations. I look at how I survived and it's like, this is what I'm living for. I want my parents to think it's okay; that I'm okay. I really like to snowboard, I like to surf, I like to do everything now that I missed out on. I'm not afraid to take a risk anymore.

I was surrounded by walls so much; every single day I was inside. It was like I was captured by something that I never wanted to happen and I think it definitely brought me to do some of the outdoor things that I love.

PATTY AND BOB: *We didn't travel for three years, and that's one of the things we really enjoyed. Now we take vacations twice a year. We make it a point to celebrate. We could be overdoing it a little. Why not?*

It's important for me to tell other people what I went through: how I made it, the different strategies of keeping hopes high and just thinking about how much you have and how lucky you are to be alive—even though this could take your life away. I've made a lot of new friends. I wanted them to know I'd been sick. I think they understood because they didn't back off. I'm not afraid to speak in front of people. I talk about the issues at school. Every kid wants more than what they have. Now I just say that I'm okay, I have what I have and I don't need more. I'm so happy to be alive and that's all that's important.

I want to be a doctor to help people out. I think I know more about the body and how it works and I know what's going on inside it. I would know what the patients are going through. I would know what's good for them. I could give them tips or advice on what to do to stay strong and not be sick. I think ten years from now I'll still want to help other kids. Nobody was there for me during my illness except my parents, but nobody was there who had been through it.

In a way, I think cancer pushed me to grow up faster than I needed to, but I'm trying to be who I am, and I'm a kid. I should be a kid while I have a chance. I don't want to get ahead of myself. Some days I want to be an adult and do those things my parents won't let me. But then I want to stay a kid, because I've already learned a lot of things that maybe an adult wouldn't even know.

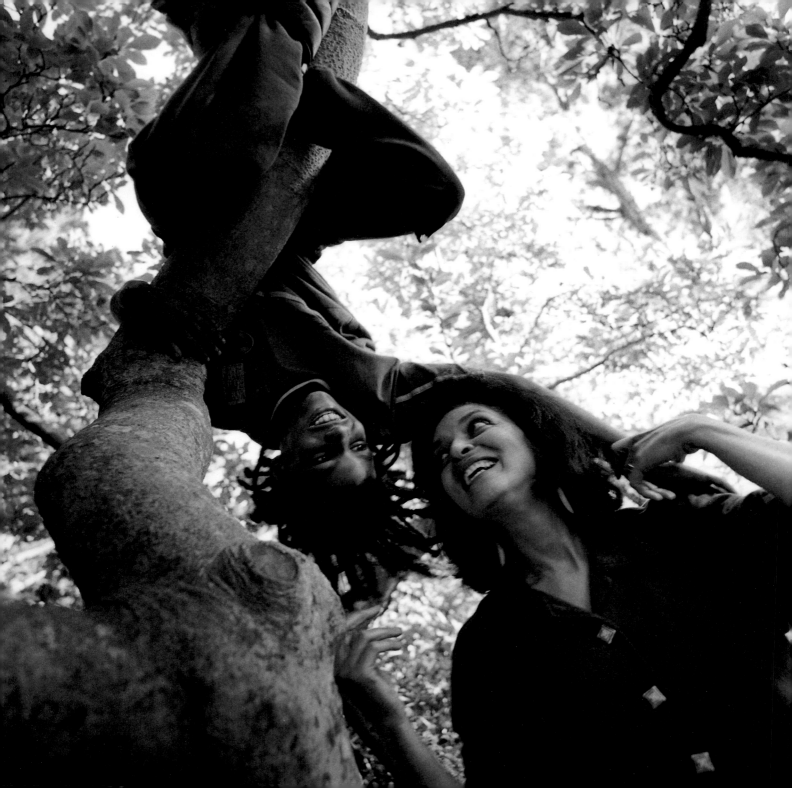

Vanetta McGee

TWENTY-FIVE-YEAR
SURVIVOR

BREAST CANCER,
HODGKIN'S DISEASE

WHEN I was a freshman at San Francisco State University, I was involved in the Black Student Movement. It was a very exciting, heady time but periodically, out of the blue, my neck would swell up and I would disappear into my bedroom and stay there for two or three days.

Finally I went to a doctor, who took one look at me and said he'd have to do a biopsy. My world stopped. I dropped out of college. I thought, "If this ain't a bitch. I'm watching my whole future being snapped up and torn away from me." I was reacting to the unknown with total fear. I was alone. I thought, "What do I do now?"

I was diagnosed in 1963, at the time they realized that radiation could help cure cancer. They gave me more rads than they should have but it saved my life. Because I was young and enthusiastic, I became a guinea pig. My doctor said he would take care of me and that we would see it through together.

While reading a *Time* magazine, I found a tiny article about the mind/body/spirit connection and it resonated for me. I already had a strong spiritual connection. I was raised in the church but I was angry as hell. In fact, I was so angry at God that I stopped praying. I remember thinking, "I'm not going to pray to you, God. I'm not going to ask for anything. I don't even know if You exist now." I got through the whole treatment and they say that if I didn't die within the next thirteen years, I'd be cured. The day I left the hospital it was raining and overcast. The minute I opened the hospital doors, it was as if Zarathrustra spoke. The clouds parted, the sun came down, and it took me straight to my knees. I knew then there was a God. And I was so grateful that He or She hadn't given up on me. My faith was back in place.

What I have learned is that my life is a tightrope. If everything is balanced, I'm okay. All I have to do is look at the scars on my body to know.

There was so much I wanted to do but I didn't know how much time I had. I thought, "Let me be fearless and go for everything." I remember making some very real decisions then. I thought I'd never get married. I said I'd never have kids. Now I realize that I said those things because I thought I was damaged goods, that no one would ever want me. This belief gave me the permission to hurt a lot of people. Cancer gave me permission to do whatever I dared to do. And I dared a lot.

When I was young and first diagnosed, I needed discipline. No one ever said *no* to me, especially when I had cancer. But I really felt that I was dealing with it the best way I knew how, which was, "I'm going to live my life to the hilt because if something does happen, I'll have no regrets."

I believe that each time I got cancer it was because of a loss of love. The first time, was when I was seventeen and my boyfriend didn't want me anymore. I was devastated, but I hadn't been taught to express emotion. Later, I fell in love with another fellow and we were going to get married. When I found out he'd been having an affair, I was devastated. Soon after that, I found a lump in my breast. That was the one place I wasn't protected when I'd had my previous radiation.

When I found the lump, I went into a deep meditation and God spoke to me. God said, "Well, Vanetta, you did it again, you got out of balance. You're a good kid so I'm not going to kill you, but you are going to have to pay a high price." When I came out of the meditation I was calmer, because I knew I wasn't going to die. When they told me it was a bilateral and they'd have to take both breasts off I said, "Okay, take them." It was then I realized that my physical self is not who I am. I am total spirit. I knew I had to let the fear go or I wasn't going to heal. The way I took care of myself, the things I ate, meditation, all these things helped me get back on my feet. That was fifteen years ago.

I have had an issue with time. I didn't know when my time was going to run out, so I didn't ever take it into thought. I never planned for anything. I can't even tell you when I was married. I don't know when I was in the hospital or when I started acting. Cancer changed my sexuality too. I'd been pretty wild. I was out all the time. But then that changed. For a year I was celibate. I'd go on dates, that was all. I didn't want a new relationship to know my story. I couldn't look at myself either. I had my breasts reconstructed very quickly, but I've had to redo them several times. One time they hardened, another time they broke. The last doctor thought he was doing me a favor by putting in bigger implants than I wanted. I don't want another operation; I just want to do my yoga and workouts.

I'd always felt that I could never—should never—have a child because I'd had so much radiation. We started the adoption process. I was working and suddenly I found out I was pregnant. I was shocked. My whole life had been an obsession about myself. I was forty-two and it was time for something else to come into my life. My son is a miracle. I am blessed.

What I have learned is that my life is a tightrope. If everything is balanced, I'm okay. All I have to do is look at the scars on my body to know. I spend so much time now staying upright and in balance. I was so young when I first got cancer, I never had any hopes and dreams. I just took what life gave me. But now I want to know what it means to have hopes and dreams. I know I am the person I am because of all of my experiences. I don't fear death because I've been close to it—twice. Death, hah! We will have to fight on that one.

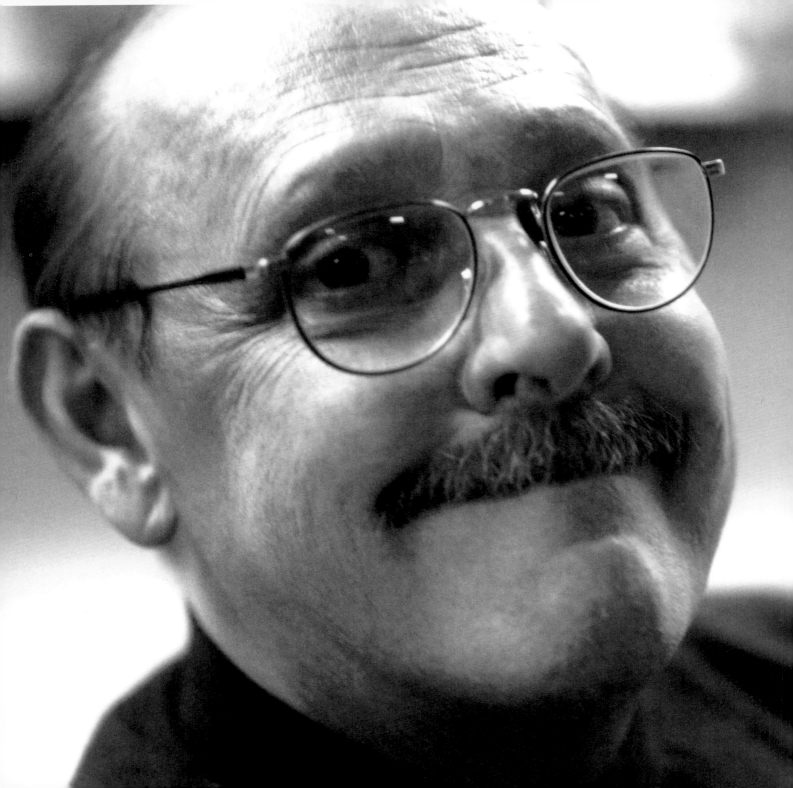

Robert Galgay

THREE-YEAR SURVIVOR
LUNG CANCER

◼

*T*HEY FOUND the lung cancer Friday the thirteenth. They radiated my brain and my chest, and I did six treatments of chemo. I've had nothing since, not even an aspirin. It didn't go away. It's still in my lung, but it's not doing anything. I see the doctor every three months. And I feel fine.

I took the cigarettes and threw them out the same day. I had been smoking thirty-five years. They haven't said that smoking causes cancer, but I know that's what it was. My sister died from lung cancer also, the year after I was diagnosed.

My wife had tried to make me quit cigarettes since we were married and I was just stubborn. When I got diagnosed with cancer I was pissed. I said, "Why me?" And I knew "Why me." I did this to myself. One of my sons smokes and he won't quit. His aunt died, there's me, his cousin. I say, "You see the hints? It's in the family, buddy." I keep talking to him about it.

I'm looking forward. Ask me a year ago to get my teeth fixed and I'd go, "Why? I'm gonna die." Now, I'm changing my attitude. I'm getting my teeth fixed. I bought two new automobiles. Me and my wife have been to St. Martin's once, St. Croix twice, and we went on a cruise to Bermuda. Before, I worked and we never found time.

I worked for Sears and Roebuck for thirty-six years. I was manager of the men's store in Burlington, Massachusetts. My oncologist told me that stress can kill you, and I was getting a lot of stress with Christmas and deadlines and all that stuff, so I said, I'm going to retire. Now I go to Sears twice a week just for coffee with the girls. It gives me therapy—I'm not missing a thing. I feel much better now that I don't have the stress.

I joined the Y. Never exercised before. But we do it faithfully every two days, and thank God for my wife, we push each other on that. It's good for the both of us.

I make goals for myself. My son's wedding—I'm going to be here for that. The Patriot season in September. I draw on stupid things.

I've gained thirty pounds since being diagnosed. I'm fighting cancer—I don't care if I'm chubby. I'll cut down on desserts, but I'm not going on a diet. I'll enjoy life as it is; I'm not going to deprive myself of things I like. Life is more fun now.

My sister Kathy, who died of lung cancer, brought me to the Wellness Community. What I get from it is the knowledge that I'm not alone with this disease, and it's interesting to see how people handle it and what they're doing. I keep it all in one room. It's my territory. There are tough times, but there are a lot of fun times in that room, too.

The support group also helped me out because, after I heard other people talk about depression, I thought, "That sounds like me." So I went back to my psychologist, who I haven't seen in ten years, and he helped me through that. I also go to the psychologist the week before I go to the doctor. That's when I usually get anxiety—about ten days before I go.

Toughest thing for me to do was, we got graves; got my grave under an elm tree. When I drive by, I don't look in the cemetery, I just look straight. No matter what happens, I've got both bases covered: I converted to Judaism just before I got married and was bar mitzvahed with my oldest son. I was raised Catholic, confirmed by Cardinal Cushing.

My oldest son always says to me, "I love you, Dad." My youngest? He doesn't say that. I keep telling him, "I love you, Chad, I really love you." My wife tells me it's hard for him when I go to the doctor. But he's one of those macho boys, you know; can't show your emotions, but I know he loves me.

I tell people to keep fighting; it's a hard disease. There will be a cure someday for it, so hang in there. Enjoy life. Have a good time, do the best you can and don't feel sorry for yourself. That's what I'm doing.

My wife's at the computer all the time. Anything comes up on TV, she goes in and pulls all the information from it. One day I may just jump on a trial, but right now I'm not thinking about it. You can overdo it, too, and keep on looking and looking and looking and not enjoy life.

I never thought about my retirement like this, having so much fun. I thought I'd probably work 'till I was seventy and I probably would never have enjoyed it at that age. Since this happened I took advantage of it. I'm retired and I'm living the good life.

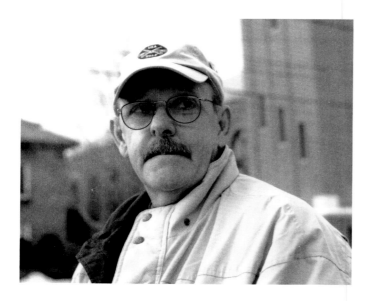

Ask me a year ago to get my teeth fixed and I'd go, "Why? I'm gonna die." Now, I'm changing my attitude. I'm getting my teeth fixed. I bought two new automobiles. Me and my wife have been to St. Martin's once, St. Croix twice, and we went on a cruise to Bermuda. Before, I worked and we never found time.

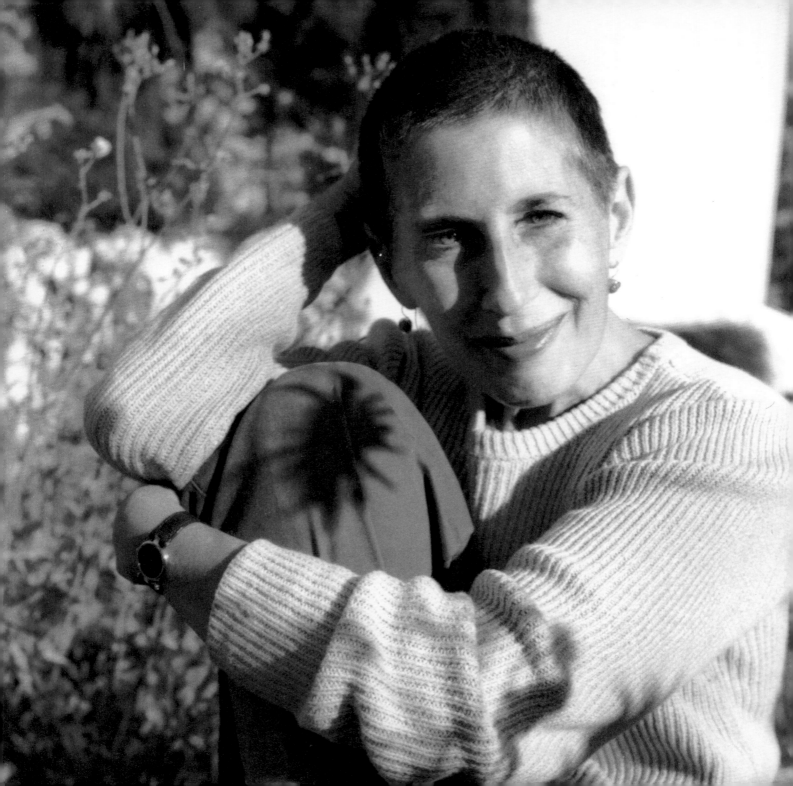

Barbara Tropp

EIGHT-YEAR SURVIVOR
OVARIAN CANCER
■

A FATAL DISEASE is one of the great levelers. I'm equal parts control freak and Buddhist. I have known since I was a child—certainly since my mother died of cancer when I was a child—that life is a crapshoot. I was totally shocked by my diagnosis of ovarian cancer. I felt that I'd never been so healthy in my life. It hit me like a ton of bricks, but I put my head down and started working to get through it. What I saw at the end of the tunnel was not death. I saw life.

I'd always been a well person. I'd never taken any drugs. I didn't even take aspirin. The most dramatic thing I'd had were fillings as a kid. That was it. I certainly had a view of mortality because my mother died when I was young and I'd lost so many of my friends to AIDS. But I felt full of life. And, fortunately, still do. One of the huge learning experiences of these years is to hold life in one hand and death in the other. And to try to balance them.

If you are diagnosed with ovarian cancer you don't get very happy by reading. I found myself totally flipped out by what I read, but I was very lucky. I had a team of five doctors, was blessed with a fabulous marriage, and I'm very close to my sister, so I felt wonderfully well supported. After my first diagnosis, I went into a short-term remission, then had a horrendous recurrence. I was running away from the thought that I could ever have a recurrence. I was doing Chinese medicine very intensely. I was brewing daily herbs. I had weekly acupuncture. Was doing Chi-gung. I felt I was safe, but I was submerging my terror that something could happen.

The tumors had come back quickly and ferociously, but I was lucky. The drugs started working. There was a point where I was certain that I was dying, just before my second surgery. I was sure my end was right near. When they opened me up, miraculously, there were no tumors there. I came back to life.

One thing I've learned through this process is to make clearheaded quality-of-life choices. I think that kicked in the moment I opened my eyes and learned that I had cancer. For some people, cancer changes their life. For me, it changed my death. I'm a pretty levelheaded person. I've always been deeply involved in Eastern thought and Chinese studies, which have been a lifeline to my soul since I was a teenager.

I was never a self-destructive person. When you are a well person, dealing with your death is a very philosophical thing. It's very easy to be a Buddhist when you are a well person. When you are a sick person and facing your death, it only then becomes clear what is really important. It's like faking a dive from the high dive. Until you are pushed off the end of the board and on your way down, you don't know how it feels. You can't know death until you have been there. I've not been there, but I've been off the board. Lucky for me, I had a bungee cord.

Because I lost my mother at a young age, I've never been one to look at life as long, long term. I wasn't married until late. I've never had my own children. I'd never had a significant relationship until recently. My life had been very similar along a continuum, except that I went from being a student to being a successful businessperson.

What shocked me was the fullness of the realization that there were only two things that mattered to me: my husband and my stepchildren. I was surprised that it was so simple.

I got ferociously angry when well-meaning people would say, "I'm sure dealing with cancer has been so difficult, but it must be a wonderful thing in many ways." There is nothing at all wonderful about this. It's disgusting. You wouldn't wish this on your worst enemy. Who wants this kind of awareness? The price of knowledge is oftentimes terrible. But the good thing is, one often doesn't have a choice. I think that has been the hugest lesson from this: you can't do anything. It's a crapshoot. The only control is to give up control.

The Victorian Age and mind-set still prevail when it comes to women and their sexual parts. I go into the oncologist's office and it's a psychic test. I hate the fact that the room is so crowded with women.

My health has been saved three times. The goddess Shiva dances on the wave with one foot, something in each arm; I've known that in small ways throughout my life. But to have to hold, so consciously, life in one hand and death in the other, is hard. And yet, one of the interesting and maybe terrific things about this experience is that I am not as terribly afraid of death as I was. I know now in a way I didn't before that everyone dies. How you die is the issue.

I don't think the way I lived had anything to do with my cancer. The cancer is in me because of my genes. I rather suspect that the way I've lived my life has helped with this. I take no responsibility for having cancer other than the fact that I'm my mother's daughter. There is a measure of comfort in knowing that I won't pass this on, as it was passed on to me and my sister.

I'm not sure that, when they discover why cancer happens, there won't be a huge, collective sigh of relief from the people that need to thrust guilt upon themselves. I feel responsible for my wellness. I don't feel responsible for my illness. Dealing with cancer is enough without dealing with the burden that you had something to do with it. If I saw Bernie Siegel, I'd pop him between the ears.

We can control so much in life now, but this is just something we can't control. I'm sure when tuberculosis or polio came around, people thought they were tying their shoes the wrong way. I have clarity that I am not responsible. Nonetheless, if you want to better your chances, what do you do? One of the things that cancer has meant to me is that I eat a great deal more meat in my diet than I used to. I think the number of hamburgers I've had in my grown-up life might have been two. Me? Chinese cook? Noodles, rice, vegetables? I taught myself how to cook because I couldn't stand the way we ate meat in this culture. I will merrily trip out to the butcher now and buy the biggest pork chop I can. I eat it with a smile on my face. Does it make a difference for anyone other than me? I doubt it. I've seen people survive who eat only potato chips.

I do what makes me feel good. And I've learned how to do that without guilt. But it doesn't make me feel good to stay up past ten at night. It doesn't make me feel good to say yes to something that, professionally, I don't feel sure about. I'm much more lax to stretch myself. My husband, Bart, has been partly responsible for that. He's been a fabulous curb on my more typical urges to exhaust myself.

I grew up always thinking that my mother had died from breast cancer. My sister found my mother's tumor records from the hospital where she died. It was very clear that she'd died of primary ovarian cancer. A year later, my sister decided to have her ovaries removed, against her doctor's wishes. The pathology came back cancerous. She said, "So you have to have this surgery now." I had started an international group for women chefs and the next morning I was supposed to get on a plane for a meeting. I called my oncologist from the plane and made plans to have surgery.

My doctor went in to remove the ovaries and saw tiny tumors scattered throughout the area. I was always somebody who thought I knew my own body. I don't know bullshit. When I had cancer, I felt fabulous. When there was no more cancer in my body, I felt terrible. I know my body but I didn't know I had cancer. When I had my most recent occurrence, I looked and felt fabulous.

I opened my restaurant, China Moon, in 1986. I lived at the restaurant. Several years later, at the time of diagnosis, I was running the business and struggling to delegate responsibilities. I was starting my organization for women in the industry. I was also beginning to have a life outside of the restaurant. I was in a high peak of activity. I loved my life.

While I was dealing with the heavy-duty cancer stuff, I was working to sell the restaurant. There was a huge amount of attending to, and it was of great concern to me. Finally it sold. What was very clear at that time was that the sale had nothing to do with my life or my death; I was simply trying to wrap up a situation so I would not leave Bart with a bloody mess. I'm a nutty Virgo, I always want to clean up. I made a will. That's very hard stuff to face.

Now, quite amazingly, I'm busy as can be consulting, writing articles, teaching. I am doing what I did before the restaurant, juggling many things and loving the diversity of it. One of the huge differences is that my family, and my extended family, is key. That's where the energy goes.

I have the great good fortune of being a very conscious person who married a very conscious man. I didn't have to learn, once I was hit by this trauma, how to start living my life or how to start having a relationship with my partner. I had cancer but I had every blessing: I was financially stable with great health insurance, I had a great marriage, I had supportive friends, I was open with my husband. I've tried to see all these blessings in context because it pains me that I have cancer. What more could you want?

I shut down sexually after the cancer. Dealing with healing wounds, with feeling that my body was the enemy, dealing with the effects of chemotherapy—it was very hard. There was no sex life for a long time. We cuddled. We kissed. I don't know what I would have done without his hugs. His touch is incredibly powerful for me. There is your beloved mate, wanting to be close, so when closeness through sex is shut down, it's bewildering. I felt guilt about that. I talked to him about it but, nonetheless, it's the stuff that can rip relationships apart.

I went into overnight menopause. You dry up. You are used to being this lush pond of juices and suddenly you are a dry mess. We had to be as creative as we could be! Sex is a different experience after menopause; there is an adjustment. There is no question that surgery and chemotherapy and psychic trauma had a huge impact on our sex life. Now, it's quite different. It's as it used to be. There is a depth of lovingness that has happened as a natural course. But again, it very much depends on who you are with.

It did have a big impact professionally for a while, as well. The drugs wrecked my palate. I couldn't taste! I came into my profession with my greatest advantage being my palate. It was as if I were suddenly blinded, and I was devastated. That did come back, but never to the degree that it was before. As I do it more and more now, it's better. I have to trust people to do final adjustments on dishes for me. That had more effect on me, psychically, than even the interim where sex was unwanted and difficult.

It is a very interesting and difficult experience. I feel like I found a place I trust now. Where I trust Shiva on the waves, holding death where I hold life. I still consider myself one of the luckiest ducks in the pond. I'm lucky to be aware of all that I have. Luck has saved me. Cancer has been a bitch, but I have a great life.

Barbara died of ovarian cancer shortly before the publication of this book, eight years after her original diagnosis. We felt that the way she lived her life and the power of her words could be helpful to readers of this book. She will be missed.

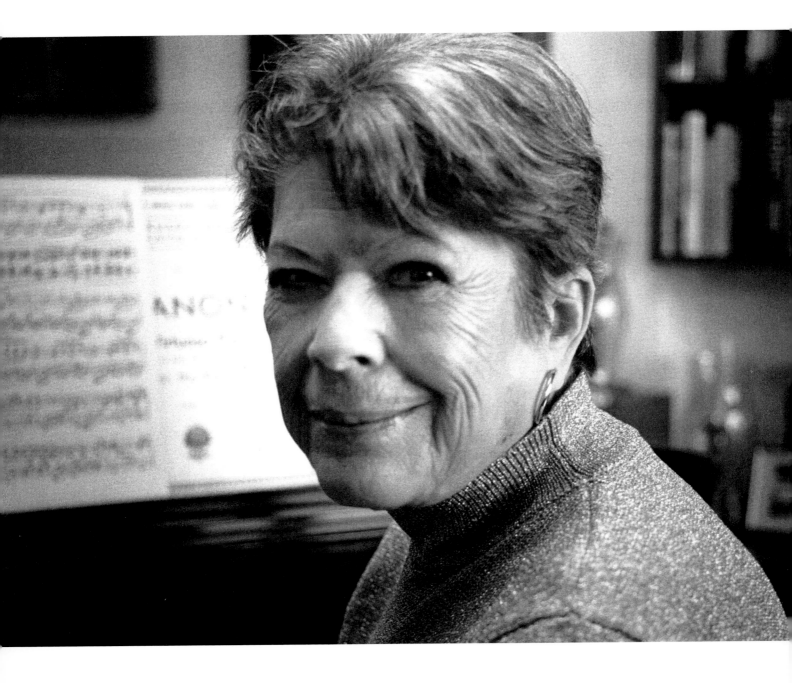

Marilyn French

EIGHT-YEAR SURVIVOR
ESOPHOGEAL CANCER
■

I COME FROM a generation where a diagnosis of cancer was a death sentence, so that's how I associated it, with death. I was sixty-two when I was diagnosed.

One morning when I woke up to go and give a speech, I went to talk and my voice sounded funny. I only had half my voice. After I consulted many doctors, it was determined I had cancer, but couldn't find the primary site. If I hadn't kept bugging the doctors to find out what was wrong, I think they just would have dropped it. One doctor said, "I think *you* know where the site is." I thought, "I do?" I went home and I thought. And I did.

The summer before, I had been sitting on my porch in the country eating a sandwich with rye bread. As the bread went down, it hit a lump and I felt it, right there in my esophagus. It made an impression but, at the time I thought, "I'm not going to think about it." I went back and told them where it was and they were able to start treatment.

I would never have called it intuition. It's not a word I use. I'm so sick of hearing about "women's intuition." Or, at least, we used to hear about it when I was young. I think it's simply awareness on a subtle level of what's going on around you. I'm a novelist; I am aware.

At the time of diagnosis, I lived alone. But I had very good friends and I had my children, who were very much a part of my deliberations. I'm not a trusting person, but the doctors were so uniformly negative that I had to think they were telling me the truth. My friends, of course, tried to be positive but they didn't lie. Nobody said, "You'll be fine," and nobody said, "It'll go away." Nobody talked to me that way. They just said, "We're here."

When I went to see the oncologist for the final diagnosis, he told me I had terminal cancer and a year to live. I blanked it completely out. I forgot it. I didn't tell a soul that it was terminal; I told everyone I had one chance out of five of living. I knew I was going to die, but I pretended I wasn't. It was a contradiction in my head, which is odd because I think I'm a very realistic person who always insists on facing the worst; facing the truth.

I write—that's what I do, professionally. But I couldn't write during almost this entire period. I couldn't concentrate on anything much. Instead, I read. I listened to music. In writing, you have to go inside, and my insides right then didn't bear looking at.

I retreated from the world when I was sick. I canceled all my speaking engagements, I saw no one except my friends. A group of my women friends—we call ourselves a coven—held meetings all the time for me when I was in the hospital, with candles. They surrounded me with their magic. Even today, we listen to each other and we talk about what's been bothering us. We laugh, we giggle, and we act like a bunch of wild women. I'm sure it helped me to get well.

You know, I really believe in a woman's world because I live in one. I probably have always lived in one, at least since I had children. The outside world makes you feel bad; degrades you and makes you smaller. A woman's world makes you bigger, calmer, more lovable and feeling loved. When my book, *The Women's Room*, made the best-seller list, I was as shocked as anyone could be, but it was a book written to get people's attention. When I finished it, I felt I had done a great thing, and I felt that I had told the truth about women in a way that had not been done before.

When I wrote *A Season in Hell* about my cancer experience, I tapped a totally different audience from my normal audience. I never wanted to be defined by cancer. I think a lot of people who read my writings don't even know that I wrote a book on cancer, and vice versa.

A Season in Hell was a difficult book for me to write. I'm not even sure why I wrote it. I suppose that I thought I was laying the disease to rest. Now, I'm very glad to have written it. I think I always write to try to understand something. I write for discovery. I discovered that I had changed. The change was inevitable and irremediable. For years, I told myself that I had to get back to where I was. By the time I finished that book, I knew that I was never going to get back to that place. I had come to feel peaceful about the new place, but I'm not sure I knew that when I started the book.

I had smoked too much and had drunk too much in my life, but I didn't feel the slightest bit of guilt about it. I enjoyed the smoking and drinking and I would do it again if I could. I never felt, "Oh, I was so bad—why wasn't I better?" I drink occasionally now, but it's no fun. In the first place, it burns my esophagus; in the second place, without a cigarette, a drink is nothing. I smoke in my dreams. I loved to smoke and I wish I could now.

I used to be more active. I was more sexual. I'm not sexual now. I had a sex life, which I don't anymore, nor do I want one. I think the chemotherapy really knocks that out of you. I traveled a great deal, but now I have great difficulty traveling by myself. At this point, I've been told that I cannot walk more than a block and I can't lift anything at all because of my heart, which was damaged by the radiation to my chest.

I used to live in the future. I used to live in what book I would finish next; in what it would accomplish, imagining that the books I wrote made a difference in the world. Perhaps they do, but a brief difference. I live much more in the moment now, which is a much healthier way to live, but it kind of eviscerates desire; it eviscerates ambition. Those things don't have any place to grow if you live in the present. They need to be rooted in long-term plans, and I never have long-term plans. It was not until several years after I recovered that I was able to say to someone, "I'll see you next year," because I really didn't think I would.

I think that when we die, we die. I don't think there's more than that. Death as a possibility wasn't horrible to me. I don't think life has any meaning at all, in the sense of some higher power giving it to me, or a meaning that stands beyond our lives. The meaning of a life is the life, and what matters in a life is what you experience—what you felt and thought and did. I felt a great deal in my life and I expressed a great deal. I had great love and still do; great pleasure as well as great pain, and I had lived. It was enough, and I could die. I made up a living will. I had long talks with my children. I told them what I wanted them to do for me. I told them how much I loved them.

A Season in Hell was a difficult book for me to write. . . . I write for discovery. I discovered that I had changed. The change was inevitable and irremediable. For years, I told myself that I had to get back to where I was. By the time I finished that book, I knew that I was never going to get back to that place.

As long as I can, I'm going to go on writing and enjoying my life as I do. Life is full of pleasures, among which writing itself is probably my greatest one. I was not aware of pleasure as much until I got sick. When you're sick, pleasures are very few and far between and you look for them—you have to almost manufacture them. When I was sick, I had a bedroom that overlooked Central Park, and if I sat up in bed I could see the sun coming up over the east side of New York City. That was a pleasure.

I thought of myself as a survivor before cancer. I mean, you *survive* life, and I've had a pretty painful one. A very rich one in many ways, but full of emotion. I'm a witness to the past and I'm here. I don't think of myself as a victim of cancer, although I think women are victimized in general by laws, by customs, and by men.

I've gotten used to thinking I'm going to live, and when something suddenly happens, like the chest pains I've been having recently, reminding me that I may not, it's a shock, and I'm upset about it. It's amazing that I've lived eight years—really amazing. So, I should be very grateful that I've had what I've had. I am, but I manage to forget.

One thing I never could tolerate is the notion that you "make war" against cancer or drugs or another disease. That's nonsense. You maybe survive it, but you don't fight it. You really don't have control, and the war metaphor suggests you do because, of course, we have to believe we control every minute. I would like to see that vanish, but it won't. People will say to me, "You beat it." And I say, "Oh no. I *survived* it."

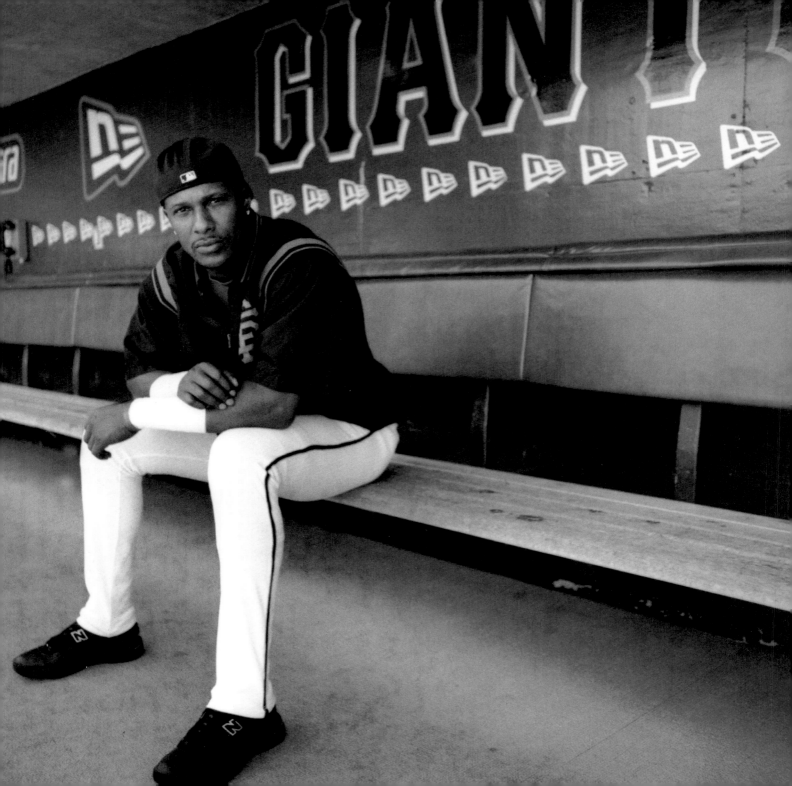

Eric Davis

FOUR-YEAR SURVIVOR
COLON CANCER

*A*T FIRST I was misdiagnosed with an abscess. I went for a second opinion and the doctor did a colonoscopy immediately. He told me I had cancer on a Wednesday, and on Friday I had surgery. It really didn't weigh heavily on my head because it was a relief to know what it was, and I could take care of it. Right after the surgery, he told me he'd gotten it all. I didn't really have time to contemplate it being cancer and it being in my body.

Chemo is poison, but the doctor thought it was right for someone my age, with my size tumor. A friend of mine, his wife is an herbalist and she cooked up some teas that I took after and before chemo. I was only down a day or two after the treatment. I wouldn't let it beat me or get me down. I can't say if that was because I'm an athlete—I would have to think that my physical condition had something to do with my tolerance, though. My muscles didn't break down.

I would look in the mirror and tell myself I couldn't be selfish: I did that for my family, other patients and people who might be in the same situation who would see me quit. I didn't want them to say: "If he quit, I can quit."

I don't think about having cancer all that often now—just when people ask me how I'm feeling. But when I'm not asked, it doesn't weigh on my mind at all. But I don't take anything for granted. If there is anything I want to do, I do it. That's different from before. I would put things off, but now if I want to say or do something, I do it right then and there.

Going to the hospital and seeing all the little kids who had cancer did something to me. I asked myself what the reason was that I got well. What would my calling be? And I thought it was to get information out about colorectal cancer and to spread the joy of being alive.

I started the Eric Davis Foundation because I wanted to raise money for colon cancer research and pediatric oncology. By me raising money, I'm able to help kids who don't have money to get treatment. That's what some of the money from the foundation does. It's not for one particular hospital—I spread the wealth. I also have an Eric Davis Laboratory at Johns Hopkins, where they do research. This is my way of paying back for my life.

I've been playing baseball for thirty years. I started when I was nine and I've played all over: San Francisco, Baltimore, Cincinnati, Detroit, and L.A. You get used to the moving around. I've been playing pro baseball for five years after my treatment. I think that, after my diagnosis, the guys on the team became more sensitive and together with their families. A man of my status and age and physical condition being struck was a wake-up call to them.

I played baseball while I was on treatment. I've developed a high pain threshold from playing sports all these years, and I was always tired from playing anyway, so I didn't see a reason why I couldn't keep it up.

I didn't like chemo. There were times when I'd be driving to the doctor's office to get the treatment, and I wanted to turn back. I didn't want to do this any more. I could smell it and it would make me sick. Sometimes, I still smell it.

It was because of my wife and kids that I kept it up. I have two girls: fifteen and eleven. My wife explained what was going on to them, and they probably heard it on TV. I didn't have a choice if people knew about it from the media. I didn't care about that, though. My job was to get healthy and to get the best possible care as quickly as I could. I would look in the mirror and tell myself I couldn't be selfish: I did that for my family, other patients and people who might be in the same situation who would see me quit. I didn't want them to say: "If he quit, I can quit." I'm part of that cancer fraternity. When you're a part of that fraternity, you have a certain obligation to be the best you can be and keep on fighting.

I feel connected to cancer through the things I do. People that I would never, ever have imagined meeting say thank you, or that they read my book and it was inspirational, or they commend me for doing the things I've done and say it helped them keep going. When I hear those things, it makes me feel that I've done the right thing.

I didn't need to draw on my faith when I was sick, because I never stopped believing. I know that I got prayers from a lot of people. God never gives you more than you can handle. So I never asked why I got it, because I knew that if it was in me, it was there for a reason. Him sparing me was for me to do good. To spread the word, help other people. I knew what it was all about.

Something I heard from another patient has always stuck with me: "Don't ever give up." Cancer can't take my body, or my heart or my mind. Never give up. That has been my motto ever since.

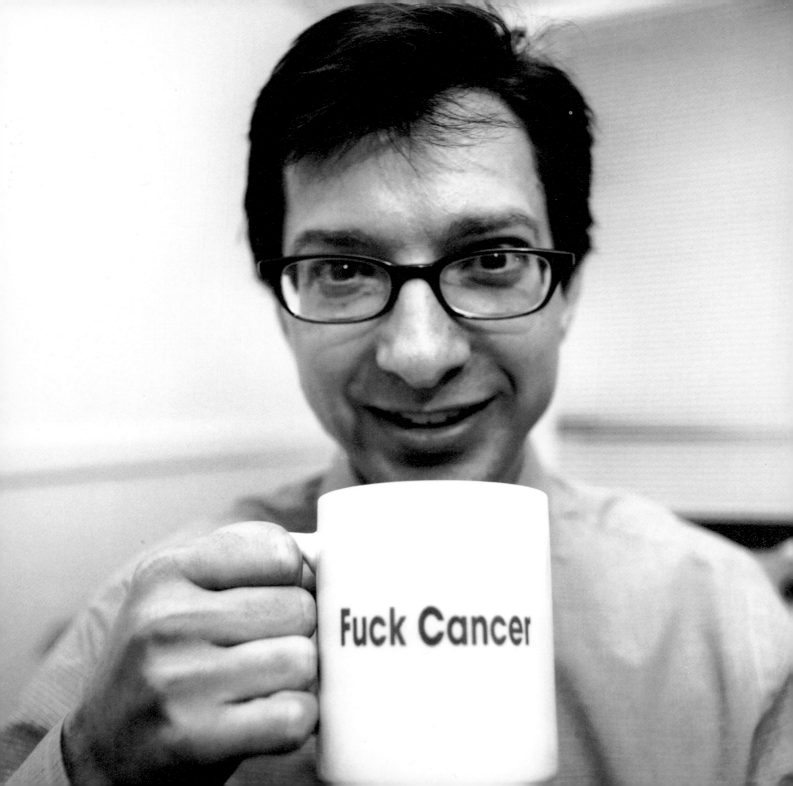

Steve Saltman

SIX-YEAR SURVIVOR
HODGKIN'S DISEASE

I QUIT TRADING on the Chicago Board of Options Exchange when I was twenty-two. I was bored and I wanted to travel, so I went into the Peace Corps. After I returned, I moved to Boston to work for a start-up forestry investment firm. While I was doing that I was diagnosed with Hodgkin's. I think of it in terms of when I got married, because I got married in November '95 and I got diagnosed March '96, four months later. It wasn't too good.

I was around thirty when I was diagnosed. On Fridays, I would work a half day and then I would get my chemo. By Monday, I was usually recovered. I walked ten blocks to the subway every day to go downtown to work. I did not stop doing that during treatment, and that helped me a lot. I walked every day, but I was so slow. My wife would make fun of me; she'd say, "You're like an old man."

I'm kind of an Internet person and I've been a computer geek since high school, so as soon as I got diagnosed I was all over the Internet and I was sending out emails. The Hodgkin's list is absolutely one of the most helpful. I found incredible camaraderie. The participants are very active and I've stayed in touch with a couple of them. It was a lifesaver.

It was important to me to know all the names of all the drugs, and to be an absolute expert. I pestered the nurses and doctors about everything that was going on. I read everything. All the books on cancer, there are a couple of tons. In the Peace Corps, there's a book they give the volunteers called *Where There Is No Doctor.* As a perverse enjoyment, I would read this book, which is a compendium of horrible things that can happen in rural medicine. I took a similar perverse satisfaction at the beginning of treatment, reading all the side effects of the drugs I was taking. I suggested to the Hodgkin's list to *not* to do research on your disease and not learn about treatment options beyond what is necessary for decision making. The side effect of every drug I took included "death."

My experience in the Peace Corps helped me with the whole cancer experience. It showed me that people everywhere have hurdles to cross, and the ubiquity of the human condition. I consider myself a Peace Corps "graduate" and also think of myself as a cancer "graduate." Survivorship is something I accomplished with the help of others, just like college or graduate school.

I decided to start a website [www.humorosis.com] to give a permanent home to my "Diagnosis + X Days" letters to my friends and to the Hodgkin's list. I kind of got into the whole vomit thing, so I added the International Synonyms for Vomit List so people could post to it. My site was very helpful to me, both as a forum for my thoughts and as a means to validate my experience. I received—and still receive—many emails from people saying that my site has been helpful in their treatment.

I started this business selling things on my site. I sold mugs that said FUCK CANCER. I've never actually had anyone complain, but some people are a little offended. I always thought if I could find hospitals that would carry them in their gift shops, I could sell millions. If you could box them in a plain brown box that says specifically, "Don't open this unless you have cancer," you might actually get it through the gift shop doors and next to the condolence cards and little inspirational angels.

I respond to stress with humor. I don't respond to depression with humor. But I wasn't depressed about my cancer. I never, ever believed I would die. Of course, my doctors told me I wouldn't die, which helped.

Anyway, I got into the whole thing but I was not able to turn it into a business. It's hard enough to have cancer, let alone start a business when you have cancer. And when I put cancer behind me, I kind of wanted to put all this behind me, too. On top of everything, I was laid off from my job. I definitely would have left sooner if I hadn't been sick, but I couldn't, because you can't get a job when you have cancer. Plus, I would have lost my health insurance.

My wife and I were just married, so my diagnosis was a big bummer for her. I told her she bought damaged goods. We'd been together for four years, so I was never concerned that she would take off or anything, but it certainly was not what she bought into, having to deal with a guy who was going to be home every weekend in bed.

I still eat ice cream and stuff. Why not? I ate a lot of Ben and Jerry's Chocolate Fudge Brownie ice cream during chemo. It was the only thing that never got marked by the chemo taste.

My wife was not a part of the Hodgkin's list. She was kind of shut out of it. She didn't get it and couldn't really participate. I didn't want her to, either. I kind of just wanted to deal with it alone, so it was very tough on her. Tougher on her than me, frankly, because I was in charge. She wasn't.

I could take control. I could say, "I am going to be sick today. I don't feel well." But she was like, "Is he going to be sick today? Is he going to want to eat anything? Is he going to come home and complain about the food I made because of the smell in the house?" Or she'd want to go out and do something and I wouldn't want to go. I think it's very hard on spouses and partners. We got through it because the treatment ended. I don't want to put any happy faces on it.

I think my wife and I have really moved on. We've had a lot of life changes since I was sick. I have a new job and we bought a house. Our financial situation has improved. We've had a kid. Having been sick definitely made me want to have kids more. I don't know—perpetuate the family. Bigger-issue stuff. No longer just money and beer. I can't get life insurance but, being a business-oriented guy, I solved that problem by buying a house that has rental units in it, so it will generate income if anything happens to me.

I have no fear that anything that I've been through affects my son. None. I don't think my disease was genetically involved. I hitchhiked all over Africa. I traveled in Russia for six months. I've been almost everywhere and I've had all kinds of horrible illnesses. I think the cancer was from something that I did traveling. So I don't associate my cancer with anything ongoing or anything I can pass on to my kid.

Now, I really try not to eat a lot of red meat. Well, I *try* not to eat a lot of stuff, but I eat it anyway. I still eat ice cream and stuff. Why not? I ate a lot of Ben and Jerry's Chocolate Fudge Brownie ice cream during chemo. It was the only thing that never got marked by the chemo taste.

I was far more open about having cancer than anyone I know. I don't want to say that I wore it on my sleeve, but maybe I did a little bit. Played the cancer card to get in front of lines. My wife and I used to make jokes about that whenever we were at the movies. She'd say, "Tell them you have cancer. I don't want to wait any more."

Some people say cancer made them think more deeply and calmly. Not me. It's probably made me more impatient, because who wants to waste their time with bullshit? That said, I think I went through a period where I was different and now I'm back to where I was. Maybe that's because the disease was a year of difficulty and then it was gone. I didn't spend a single night in the hospital; I was never at death's door. I had constipation that would kill a person, but I was closer to death when I had malaria in Africa.

I wondered if I didn't get out of it what other people got out of it. I don't think cancer has made me a better person. I'm still kind of an asshole sometimes. Kind of a sarcastic prick. I was then and I am now. Should it have changed me? I don't know. I mean, it does change you because everything changes you, but I can't point to some specific element, except that I have a scar and I get nauseous at the mention of certain foods. Maybe I compartmentalize, but I don't even sympathize as much with other people who have illness. I feel for them. I know what they're going through because I've been there, but I don't know that I'm any more caring.

I've actually felt guilty because I do sometimes wish that I'd changed. They say that if it doesn't kill you it makes you stronger. I do think it's made me stronger because you carry with you your successes and I handled treatment well. I went to every chemo, I took my radiation,

I took my medicine, I was a very good patient, and I'm now cured. So hopefully I'll become a better investment banker one day.

My website is a way to tell people not to fuck with me because I've beaten cancer. If you're doing business with me, you'll find out. I've met CEOs of big companies—billionaires—and I've done something they can never do. That works in business. Maybe that's one reason I tell certain people—to get an edge in sort of an opportunistic way. Like a twelve-year-old boy who talks about the cuts he got. Maybe I still think that way. Maybe it's a male thing. Maybe I'm wacko!

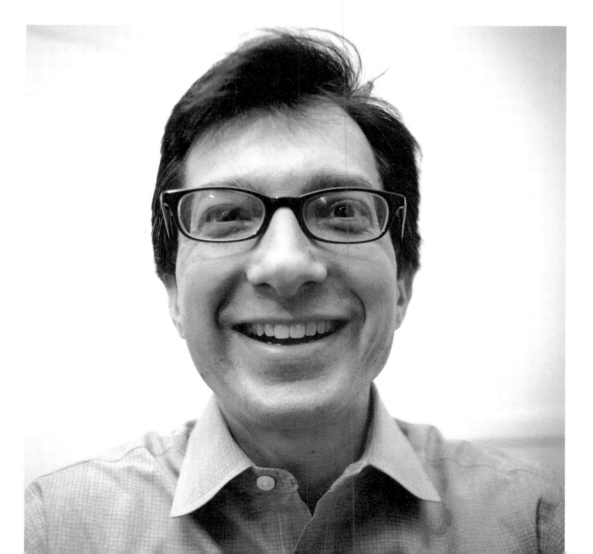

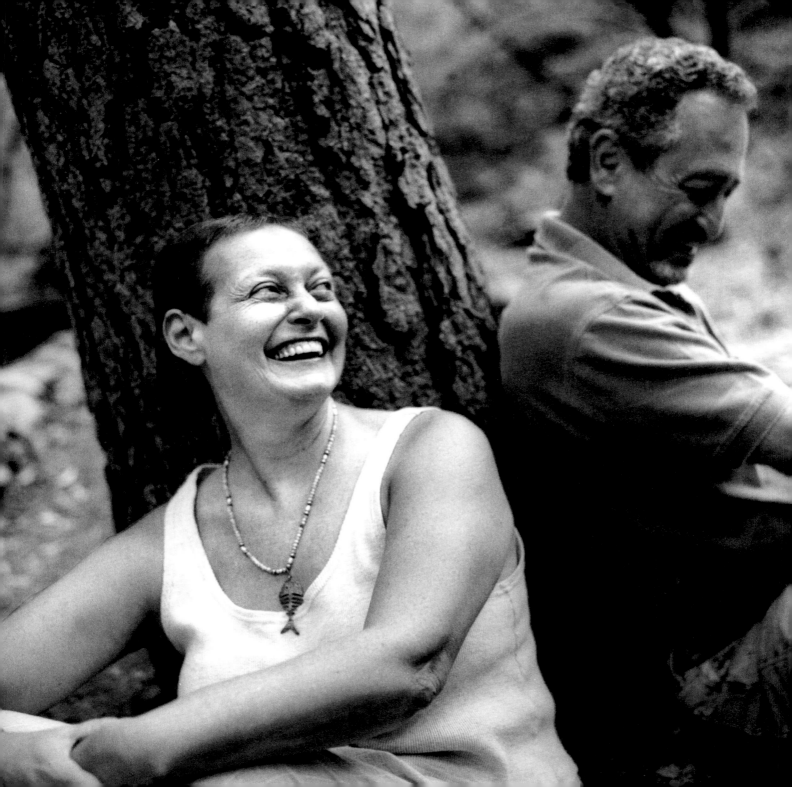

Carole Hart

SEVEN-YEAR SURVIVOR
BRAIN AND LUNG CANCER

*A*T THE TIME I was diagnosed, the word workaholic characterized me most accurately. I took myself and my work—producing movies for film and television—very seriously. I would become obsessed with my projects, and get deeply hurt and angry when others didn't consider them as important as I did. My social life, if I had any, was built around my colleagues on the film I was making. People would be close for a very short time, then everyone would disperse when it was over. I had other friends. But I never saw them and rarely spoke with them.

Just prior to getting diagnosed, I was flying around the U.S. and Canada, working eighteen hours a day on three major projects in three different cities. I had been a heavy smoker and had started again after quitting for a year and a half. I was really abusing myself. I was approaching my fiftieth birthday when I started feeling funky. I ignored it. At one point I blacked out completely in the middle of a phone conversation. Eventually I went to a doctor, who took CAT scans of my chest and head, which showed I had lung cancer that had metastasized to my brain.

Soon after that, I got a phone call from a film editor I'd worked with who told me about a medicine man in South Dakota who had healed people with cancer. I was interested. I was on the mend and I wanted some insurance.

I didn't want anyone to know, so I pretended I had "female problems"—that usually ended the discussion and it didn't sound too life-threatening. When I went into the hospital for a biopsy, I was in a very powerful state of denial. After the biopsy, the neurologist came into my room and said things looked grim. He told me I had three or four months left; that they didn't hold much hope for me because the lesions in my brain were scattered all over the place and therefore inoperable, and chemotherapy couldn't get to my brain.

We saw many other doctors, all of whom were telling me I wasn't going to make it. I got angry. Very angry. I've always had trouble with authority figures. I just wasn't going to let them be right. The willfulness and obstinacy that I'd suffered from all my life were suddenly life saving.

I was led to a doctor who had pioneered the work on taxol and ovarian cancer, and was now experimenting with taxol and lung cancer. He thought it might keep me alive for a few more years. I went for it because I didn't have any better offers. I also began working with a gifted nutritionist who used natural substances—food, juices, and supplements—to sustain my immune system and counter the toxic effects of the chemo. I did deep-tissue massage to further eliminate toxins from my body, acupuncture to create a clear channel for healing energy, and visualization and hypnotherapy to deal with emotional and psychological issues in my life that might have contributed to my illness. In doing so, I finally had to look at the profound

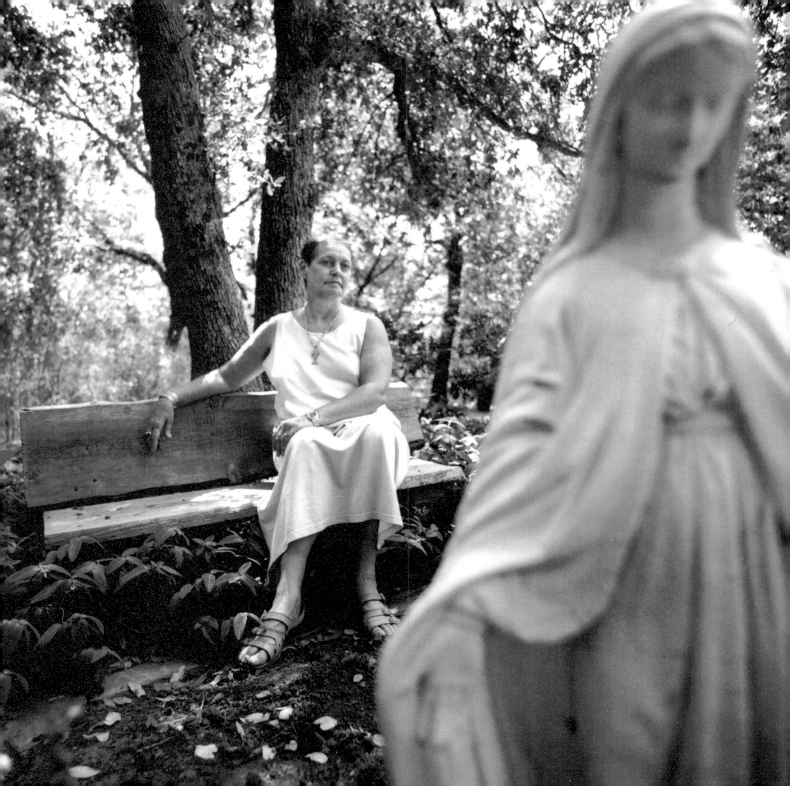

ambivalence I felt about being alive. I saw that I was addicted to my work because the only way I could justify my existence was by giving back big-time—as big-time as I could manage. I had to stare down my negativism. I had to shift my way of looking at things. I had to make an affirmation: "I want to live."

One night while dining with friends in a restaurant, my temperature shot up from normal to 105, while my blood pressure was radically dropping. By the time I got to the hospital, the doctor told my husband, Bruce, that I was dying. I held on as tightly as I could to Bruce's hand until I couldn't hold on any longer. I let go. As my fingers uncurled and I felt myself falling away, it seemed as though a grand-sized hand slipped under me and held me here. I woke up two days later in the ICU. They thought I had pneumonia, but I knew that I'd survived a healing crisis—a time when so much of the cancer suddenly breaks up that it's toxic to the system. They took X-rays of my chest and discovered that the tumor in my lung was half the size it had been just weeks ago.

Soon after that, I got a phone call from a film editor I'd worked with who told me about a medicine man in South Dakota who had healed people with cancer. I was interested. I was on the mend and I wanted some insurance.

The medicine man was Charles Fasthorse. He is a direct descendant of the famous Lakota prophet Black Elk. We made a date to meet in several months. In the meantime, I was feeling so good, I went back to work on a movie I'd begun before the diagnosis. It was a very stressful experience. Within three weeks, my lymph nodes were swollen and the tumor started to grow again. I wasn't up to the stress. It was such an amazing lesson—one I had to be taught again and again and again. Stress sucks the life out of you.

When I got to South Dakota, I had stopped the taxol because the cancer had figured out a way around it. Instead of being on the mend, I was being threatened again. Charles Fasthorse told me that what would make this healing possible was my belief in its possibility. In the Black Hills of South Dakota where the buffalo roam, it's easy to believe. In my Manhattan apartment, I knew it would be quite a lot more difficult. I prayed for a concrete sign of success that I could take back to the concrete canyons I call home.

We went into the sweat lodge at sunset. The fire had been burning since five o'clock in the morning, so it was extremely hot, and I was really scared going in. I didn't know if I could handle it. It's an endurance test, which is part of what makes it work.

Inside, we prayed for friends and relatives and ourselves. The Lakota people sitting in the circle prayed that the Spirit would come in and heal me. During the sweat, Charles said he was puzzled by what he'd seen at the bottom of my lungs: red mud moving through a sieve that looked like a peach pit. We were in there three and a half hours, singing, chanting, and tossing herbs, cedar, and water on the hot rocks. The water steamed and hissed, and the herbs crackled, and created fragrant smoke. It was very cleansing inside and out. When I emerged, I felt like I'd undergone a profound transformation on many levels.

As I was changing my clothes for the feast that followed, I noticed there were reddish stains around the neck of the T-shirt I'd been wearing. I showed the shirt to Charles Fasthorse and he gasped. On the back of my shirt there were tiny points, the color of red clay, in the shape and the size of my lung. Here was the answer to my prayer. I had something to take home with me. I felt triumph and joy on so many levels. It was one of the highest moments of my life.

I take things one or two at a time now, if I can. My schedule has slowed down a lot. I'm not a workaholic anymore. I no longer have to define myself by what I do or accomplish. I also got involved with a healing community that teaches an indigenous way of life. It sustains me. I've gotten back into teaching yoga. Before my cancer, if a film project had fallen through, I would have blamed myself and gone crazy. Now I just go to a yoga class. My real work is in my growth as a person. That's challenging enough to keep me occupied.

When I got sick, it was almost like going to my own funeral and hearing the eulogies. Everybody was calling. They told me how much I'd given to them and how much I meant to them—I had no idea I'd had such an impact. People don't take the time in daily life to appreciate each other. It was overwhelming. And deeply healing. I used to be someone who just railed against the gods. Now I can mostly find my way back to gratitude.

As frightening as all of it was, I wouldn't give up a moment of the experience because I don't know which of the many moments were the teachers. I do know that I'm not so afraid of dying anymore. The moment I really experienced myself dying turned out to be blissful. That makes me feel like, whatever death is, it's not going to be the end, and it's not going to be awful. It will be a transition to a new place and a new form. I'm certain I'll be back because I have so much more to learn that I'll never get through it all this time around. And I'm exhilarated by that possibility.

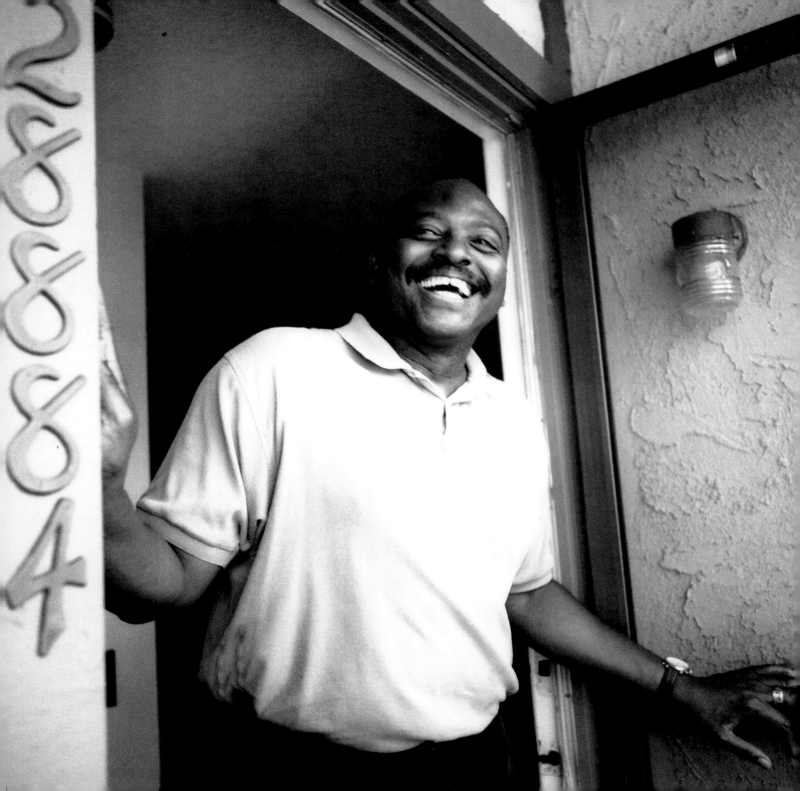

Woodrow "Woody" Brokenburr

FORTY-YEAR SURVIVOR
OSTEOSARCOMA
■

I WAS DIAGNOSED forty years ago with osteosarcoma—
a type of bone cancer. At that time, hospitals in Florida were
segregated, and I was in the colored ward. They had about
thirty-five beds, all in the basement, for everything from
infectious diseases to women having babies. They told me
that I was going to lose my leg. It was very traumatic because
I was ten years old and at the beginning of my life. I'll always
remember the night before I went into surgery. I called home
and my father told me that, before I went to bed, I should

ask God to spare my life. So I did, in my own childlike way, and I never had a fear that I was going to die. I just knew that I would be okay.

I remember the kids in my class. They all sent me letters that I kept for a lot of years. The kids were all pretty kind except for a few who harassed me and mimicked the way I walked. I recovered rather quickly with the help of my support network: my mom, my dad, my aunts. I have these two aunts who I used to go see in Ft. Lauderdale every summer. They would make me go to the beach with them, go to church—anywhere—without the prosthesis, so I just started overcoming my self-consciousness.

Dating has been a challenge. I encountered people who didn't want to go out with me because I had only one leg. That was their loss, because I always had a good time, regardless. I dance as well as anyone. I do everything.

My father bought me a bike when I was maybe twelve. I used to pedal one pedal and my cousin would sit on it with me and pedal the other pedal, and we would ride all around town. Every Sunday we did that after church. We would get on that bike and we would race and we'd go everywhere. And that's what you've got to do—just make it work and don't be afraid.

I have three kids and I love talking to them, because I think they're growing up to be wonderful individuals. I always like to hear my youngest son say, "You're a great dad." It does wonders for my heart. My ex-wife was saying that they were in an airport and he felt the need to announce that his father was a cancer survivor. He's proud of the fact that I'm moving forward and not letting it get me down.

I just kept moving forward. Every blue moon I have a pity party, but I always put a limit on it—maybe give myself a minute and then move on. I have a seven-year-old and sometimes he wants to go to the park and run around. I'm not able to chase him, and those kind of things make me feel a little sad, but I do the best I can and I think he understands that. I've always taken him to whatever I was doing in the community, so he's always seen me being active.

I've always expressed myself through volunteerism, ever since I was ten years old. I've always volunteered with the Red Cross, and when I attended university I would go to a house for juvenile delinquents and play basketball with them. I was chairman of the board of Thousand

Oaks Chamber and right now I'm working on a project with the superior court in Ventura County. Having had a disability makes you stronger. Your fiber is more intact. I want to make a difference. God has given me lots of abilities and I think you have to give back. People always gave to me, so I want to give back in return.

Recently, I've been fundraising for the American Cancer Society. I always shied away from it because I didn't want to be with cancer in my face every day. But I tried it and have been very successful. Throughout my life, I've been searching for where I should be. It appears that I'm effective in the cancer community, which is real rewarding. People see me and they know they can make it. I always believed in mentors. It's all about having an example.

My quest in life has always been to get the best prosthetic device that I could find, so that I can be mobile and do the things that I need to do. The first prosthesis I had was really heavy, made out of wood. I can remember when my father took me to get the fitting; I could hear them sawing on the wood. Now they've evolved with pneumatics, and the fit is a lot more comfortable. The insurance company is a constant hurdle; they say that I can only have one leg a lifetime. And even though I fight them and win, I tire every time I have to do it. The cost of those things has increased dramatically, and you don't get anything for wear and tear. The last leg I bought was $25,000.

I never thought much about being a forty-year survivor until recently, because I'm turning fifty. All of a sudden, I realized it's a blessing to have lived this long. I remember dreaming that I wanted to work at Price Waterhouse and live in California, and that dream has been realized. Now I would like to spearhead a philanthropic organization that directs wealthy people's funds to worthwhile causes if they don't have the time to do it themselves. Cancer would be one of the causes.

I think no matter what you're facing, you should try to find the center of your soul. I go to church. I pray every day. I meditate and take time just to be quiet. I sit under this tree and do nothing, or read a good book or sip champagne. I think that leading your life as an example is important, and I hope that my children will gain some tools by watching my life.

I never thought I would be forty years out. I probably never thought that I'd have kids, either. I just thought I'd never meet anyone that I liked or who would be strong enough to be with an amputee. It's gotta take special people to deal with that.

My father bought me a bike when I was maybe twelve. I used to pedal one pedal and my cousin would sit on it with me and pedal the other pedal, and we would ride all around town. Every Sunday we did that after church. We would get on that bike and we would race and we'd go everywhere. And that's what you've got to do—just make it work and don't be afraid.

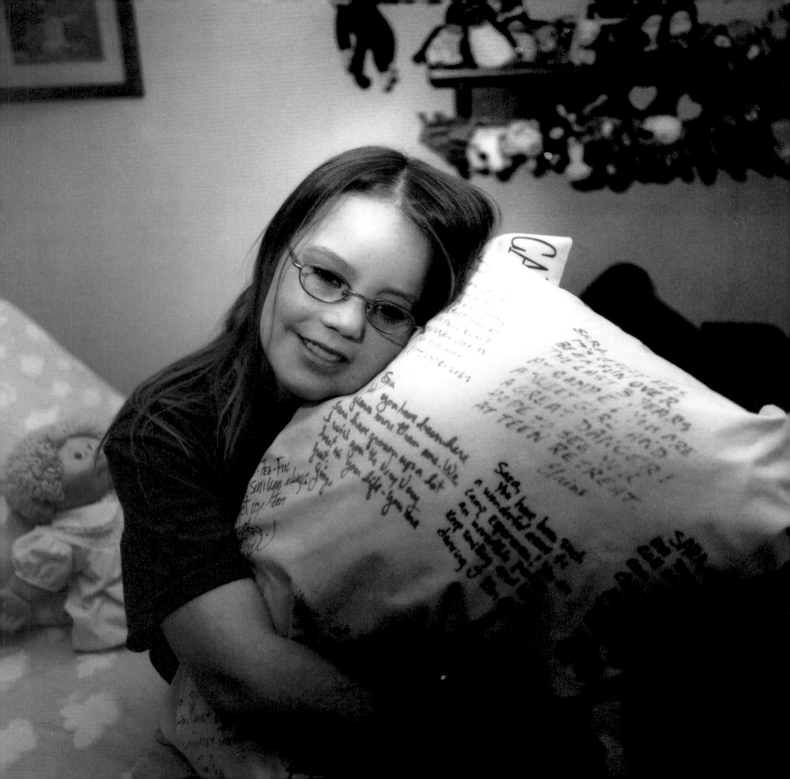

Sara Brooks

MOTHER: *Belinda Ford*

SIXTEEN-YEAR SURVIVOR
RHABDOMYOSARCOMA

■

WHEN I WENT to elementary school, kids made fun of me. Nobody was my friend. If it wasn't for my mom, I would have committed suicide.

I had radiation to my sinuses, which deformed my face. I've had lots of surgeries to reshape my face since I was two, but now it's almost totally fixed. I have a prosthesis—a glass eye. It doesn't produce tears and my lashes are all thin and it doesn't blink. That's pretty much what people were making fun of me for.

BELINDA FORD: *Over the years I just tried to point out to her that many people go through the same thing. She would always tell me, "You don't understand." I agreed with that, but I told her to look around her at the hospital and she didn't have to look very far before she found a story that's a lot worse. But she would get pretty depressed about the kids making fun of her. Of course, that would really make me mad. There was many times I wanted to go strangle some kids. And there was many times I wanted to even slap parents, too!*

Prior to her being sick, I worked in a radiologist's billing department and the ladies would always discuss how, "Man, I just couldn't handle that if that were my child" or whatever. And then when it does happen, you realize you're tougher than you think you are.

It was a long time before I got to the point where I didn't care what other people thought of me. In these last couple of years I realized it's not other people that I need to impress but God Himself. People are just kind of callous.

I met my best friend when she asked me to go to her family Bible study. When I walked in the door, I felt welcome. I felt like they were saying, "Come in; be at home." I went back the next day and kept going. I started praying, and I asked, "God, why me? Why did I have to go through this?" After a year of asking, He finally said that I would help the kids. I started raising money and I bought Hope and Halo Beanie Babies to donate to all the cancer kids at the hospital and to minister to them. I was telling them that they're not alone. And that I know what they're going through.

I went to a camp for cancer kids for eleven years, one week every summer. It's a camp for kids from six to fifteen and I used to go there and talk to other kids that had been through it and were going through it. Camp taught me to reach for my goals and work for them. And if anything tries to hold me back or pull me down, I shut it out. It's just me and my goal. I want to become a doctor. For the rest of my life, I'll help kids.

Sara was always—and still is—a very strong-willed person. She decides she wants something and she fights pretty hard to get it. We always maintained that was the reason she got through it so young was that she fought. It always took me and two or three nurses to hold her just to get a simple shot down! She had quite a reputation around the hospital when she was two years old. She was tough.

I feel that I look normal because, when I look at myself in the mirror, I'm used to it. I'm in an alternative school now instead of public school, and there's only like sixty kids in my whole school, so everybody pretty much knows everybody. There, I feel like people see me, not my face.

Sometimes people will ask me about it. A lot of them are scared; you know, they'll say, "Can I ask you a question?" and I say, "I had cancer." They're like, "How'd you know I was going to ask that?" and I say, "You're not serious, are you!" But I'm open to talking about it.

She is a little more understanding with other people now. It used to be, we'd go shopping and some little kid would stare at her, she'd be real mean and ugly because it would hurt her feelings. She would stare back at them and make ugly comments, very loud. I would be trying to explain to her, it's a little kid, they don't understand; they're just curious as to why you look like this. She was definitely boisterous about it. And there were times when I wanted to be, too, because you realize just how rude people can be.

I have one real brother, three stepbrothers, and one stepsister. My real brother is the only one that really saw me through any of it. He had to stay at home while I was in the hospital. My mom always stayed with me, so I can see why he would be jealous—I got a lot of attention and he was shoved aside.

When Sara was ill, I stayed with her the whole time and her brother, who was five or six, stayed mostly with my sister. I felt guilty leaving him at home. But Friday nights, her dad would come up and stay with her, while I would go home and pick up my son. I would usually go back up to the hospital Saturday night. My son was pretty much ignored. It was not easy.

I think he takes it out on me some. As he got older, I maybe overcompensated from feeling guilty for ignoring him during that period. But now that he's twenty-two, I'm beginning to think, okay, I've compensated, now it's time to quit!

Several months ago, he and I and Sara had our first heart-to-heart ever, about her being sick. The two of them seemed to argue constantly, and one night I'm like, this is enough. I was just tired of them bickering back and forth, never

At school dances I never danced. I was always the nerd and people would just laugh at me even more, so I just sat in the corner. But as I get older, I feel like I'm more confident. Like I said earlier, I don't care what people think about me, so I want to dance more and have fun—get my groove thing on, you know?

being nice to each other. It was pretty revealing. He really did feel ignored a lot. Since we've had our discussion, I think it's definitely triggered some love.

I like people doing things for me, you know, so I like giving back. I've been depressed before and felt like nobody cared about me. When I'm like that, I like people to come cheer me up. So I try my best to give as much as I can to other people.

I think her experience has made Sara a very thoughtful person: every birthday, every little thing that comes up, she remembers it. And wanting to do the Beanie Baby thing, which was great.

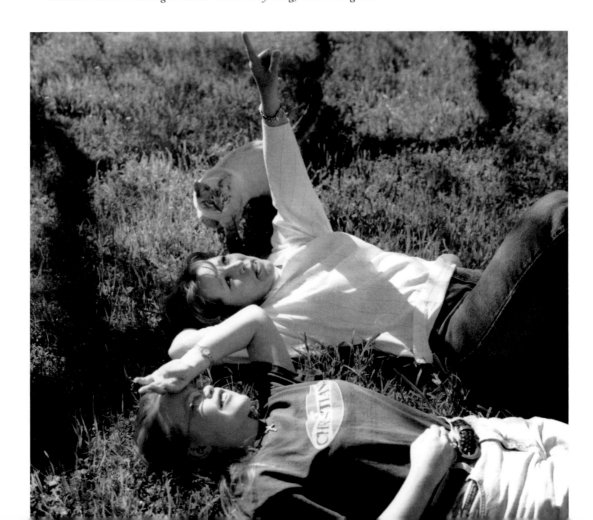

I can't wait to move out on my own. Sometimes I feel like I'm restrained, like a human being in a cage or something, and I'm trying to break out. But I was surprised when my mom let me have a car. And the dress she bought me for the prom. I mean, it wasn't like a little skinny thing, it was poofy, but the top of it came down kind of low.

It hasn't been easy to let her grow up. Driving was a big deal. My husband's the one that taught her how to drive; I was just like, "No!" It has been real hard to realize she's eighteen. Like last weekend, she comes in telling me that her and her friend are going dancing, and I'm like, "Wait a minute—I'm just not ready!" It's been difficult to let her venture out.

At school dances I never danced. I was always the nerd and people would just laugh at me even more, so I just sat in the corner. But as I get older, I feel like I'm more confident. Like I said earlier, I don't care what people think about me, so I want to dance more and have fun— get my groove thing on, you know? At the prom, me and my date were swing dancing, and he swung me around and my dress was flaring out and wrapping around me and he picked me up and did that side-to-side thing. People probably were laughing at me, because I can't dance. But I was having fun, you know?

I think I might like to have a boyfriend. I don't get depressed, but I get lonely. And it's a lonely that not just my family can fill. I see my friends go out with their boyfriends and talk about romantic dinners together and all of this and I'm like, "Okay, shut up. Don't tell me that." It's loneliness that makes me want a boyfriend, but other than that, I'm okay.

I'll be scared when Sara starts dating. The young man that took her to the prom—I was very relieved. He was very nice, very polite, very gentlemanly. Her friends have boyfriends, and the thought has crossed my mind that if Sara wants a boyfriend so bad, to what extent will she go? But when I think about it and know her, I don't think I have to worry about her being taken advantage of. I don't think she would allow that to happen.

I kind of feel things in myself more than just a regular person. When I think of my experience I think of pain, mostly. And even the kids making fun of me, that was kind of pain, too. But I feel like cancer was a preparation for things. Like maybe that was the worst part of my life, and now everything else is just no big deal.

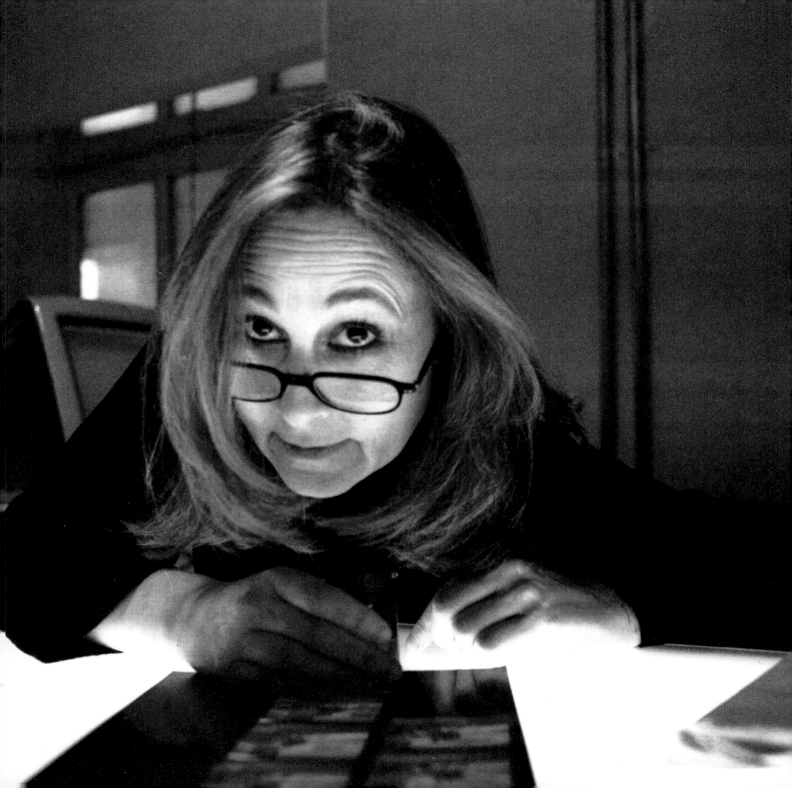

Barbara Sadick

TWO-YEAR SURVIVOR

SQUAMOUS CELL CANCER
OF THE URETHRAL
DIVERTICULUM

I AM BASICALLY an atheist, so I have never believed in miracles. I believe that what has happened to me, however, is almost miraculous. Although there has been trauma and fear, I feel extremely lucky. And though I shake each time I see my surgeon, I have thus far had no recurrence. To have survived cancer amazes me, and I realize that I cannot waste this great gift of life. I almost feel chosen.

My cancer had gone undiagnosed for some time. I was generally uncomfortable in the vaginal area, and never felt quite well. I had an IVP and sonogram, which showed a diverticulum—a lump the size of a walnut—leaning against my urethra. My surgeon took a sample from what he thought was an irritated area outside it; just routine, not thinking that anything would really be there except infection. But it was an extremely rare type of cancer.

My particular cancer had everything to do with femininity. My doctors were working on a strategy to remove a cancerous mass in a very sensitive area, keeping in mind my age and womanhood and sex life. They were several years younger than I, and knew how important feeling sexually whole was to me. I had a great fear of looking mutilated.

In order to go for a complete cure, I had to have my ovaries, uterus, fallopian tubes, cervix, and bladder removed. I was in shock. I thought that if I survived, my physical choices would make me a deformed mutant no matter what way we decided to treat it. There were plenty of stigma; removal of my bladder and catheterization through a stoma upset me greatly. This to me, at diagnosis, seemed a horror. I felt all choices were equally awful and humiliating. My entire womanhood was at stake.

I love my surgeons deeply, whereas, before, I had little respect for doctors. I credit their great skill, their steadiness, and their humanity and compassion with having saved me.

My surgeon built a new bladder, out of which my urine is emptied through an outside stoma. It's called an Indiana Pouch. This is a major life change. I catheterize once every four to six hours, so I rarely am able to sleep through a whole night. Sometimes my bladder, which is built out of small and large intestine, spurts and leaks. That has taken getting used to, and is sometimes embarrassing. They also had to cut into my vaginal tube, which required significant reconstruction and was one of the most traumatic parts for me.

Going from sickness to health was actually a progressively positive experience. I recovered rather quickly, as I was not in need of chemotherapy or radiation, although it took about five months to be able to walk normally again. Now, nobody would ever know that I have had cancer unless I told them.

People now say that I look better than I ever have, or that there is something different about me. I don't really think of myself as different today, except for the fact that I think I am stronger and have been tested. But, for the first time in my entire life, I feel special.

There is much in life that I am still looking for, and I am determined to find it. One of those things is a man who is special and mature; someone strong and understanding, who loves me in spite of my stoma. Cancer has freed me to have the kind of relationship with a man that I know I can have: a relationship that includes but transcends sex.

The experience was devastating and tough for my parents, but I think they have come to see me more clearly as I am, not as they have always thought I was. I am closer to my family and to my oldest, dearest friends, at least ten of whom I have remained friendly with for the last forty years. They gathered continually before and after my surgery to support me. I would do anything for any one of them as they have done for me. They and my family take priority over all others. My therapist has also been of the utmost importance. She helped me to express my fears and to cry and to praise myself for being strong and courageous.

Humor, and a strength I did not realize that I had, is what got me through everything. One of the most therapeutic ways of getting through this ordeal was to be able to talk about it. For much of the time I was emotionally numb, but when I finally was able to begin to process what had happened, I was compelled to talk about it all the time.

I was lucky enough to own my own photo agency with a totally dedicated, serious partner. When I returned to work, I made a point of telling each person in the office about my cancer and speaking openly about it on a regular basis. I am now able to deal with problems at work in a more even, less hysterical manner. I try to take on projects of value and with photography that speaks to me. I work with people that I like and, as a businessperson, I like to think that I am understanding and helpful and in a constant fight for my staff. They are my family, too, and it is very important to me that they be treated that way. I am willing to work less and live more, because I find that days off and trips help keep my life in perspective. Money is nice, but it is secondary.

Cancer means lots of things to me. At first it meant death, but now it means an illness that is treatable and curable if found in time. The word cancer no longer frightens me. It has awakened me to the fact that life is short and that the value of a life is living it in a principled and ethical manner. To find meaning in my life today, I need to treat people well and to be open to their predicaments and their stories. I am much less concerned than I once was about what people think of me, and am able to put things into perspective in a way I would never have been able to otherwise.

I think I can make a difference in this world by giving something back. Because my case was so unusual, I have been asked if I would allow the work that has been done on me to be photographed for further study and, of course, I have agreed to that. Also, in honor of the surgeons who gave me the gift of life, my family has set up a fund for urology research. I love my surgeons deeply, whereas, before, I had little respect for doctors. I credit their great skill, their steadiness, and their humanity and compassion with having saved me.

I feel happier more often now. I have been given a second chance at life, maybe for a purpose. Each day and each interaction means more to me than it might have. I believe I survived cancer because I am a very strong woman, from a long line of strong women. I also believe my time had not come, as I have a lot more living to do. I try to be kind and generous to others. And I continue to try to live a life of meaning. There is nothing else.

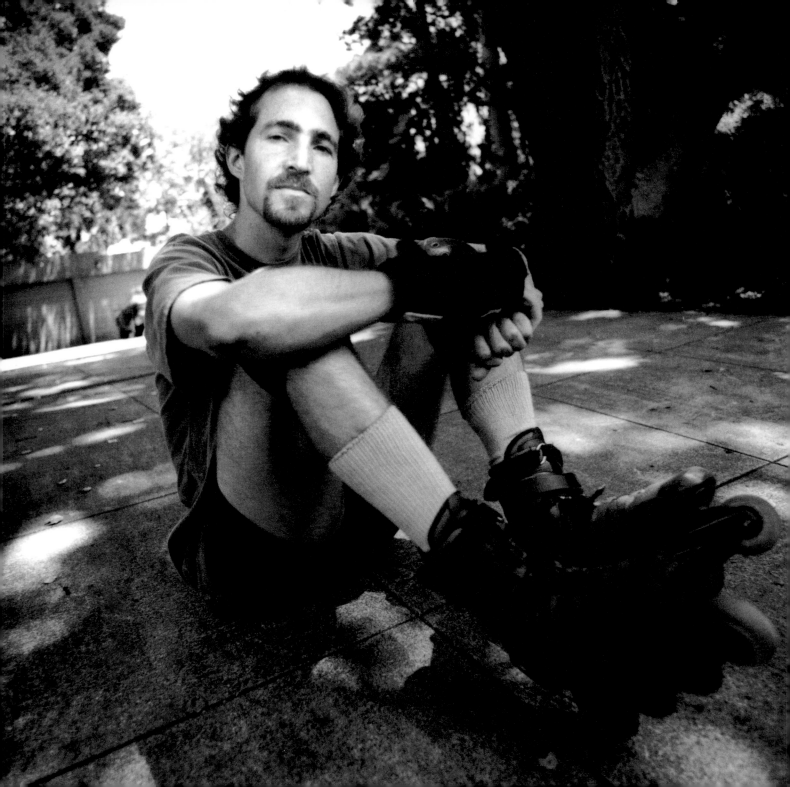

James Magee

SEVENTEEN-YEAR
SURVIVOR

LYMPHOMA

*I*N THE TWO weeks prior to Thanksgiving, I had some unusual things happen to my body: a sore armpit, stomachaches, and I was out of breath a lot. Even though I was busy in this crazy, electrical-engineering, junior-year deal at U. Penn., I still went to student health. The doctor said, "One of your lungs isn't working. You have to go to the emergency room."

Part of me was like, "What do you mean? I can't go to the emergency room. I've got work to do! I have no time. But I went and got my books and went to the ER. Eventually they admitted me and said they wanted to biopsy a lymph node.

I called my parents. This was my third year at U. Penn, and the first time I hadn't gone home to visit them in the fall. I was really stressed out from school and I was looking forward to going home for Thanksgiving; I needed the rest. I told them I was in the hospital and I didn't feel too bad, I was just having tests.

I've got an older sister and two younger siblings. They decided to come down and spend the holiday with me at school. I didn't tell them that I was having a biopsy for cancer because I was trying to convince myself that there were other possibilities.

When I got back from surgery, my whole family was in the room. We waited around for the doctor to tell us what was going on. I can remember him saying that I had lymphoblastic lymphoma. He also said that if it went untreated, I would perish within six weeks. My parents consoled me, and repeatedly reassured me they would be with me through everything. Feeling their unconditional love and support was so helpful. I really needed that. From the outset, I was determined to get better and return to the life I'd been living. I didn't allow myself to despair that I might die. I simply didn't want to hang out with those thoughts. But that determination to keep positive also disconnected me from the reality of how painful and frightening it was to be going through what I was going through. That was something I understood only in hindsight.

I've grown to feel that, to some extent, everyone who is alive is a survivor. I don't feel nearly as distinguished from people who haven't had cancer as I might have before. I've realized that life has innate, built-in losses for everyone.

I feel an awareness that it is a matter of fate that that I got this disease and survived where others did not. In some way, I have an obligation to appreciate this privilege. I don't want to forget. My life feels richer when I think about this. Part of being a survivor is this awareness that life doesn't measure out things in a fair manner. That is a sobering, often challenging thing to accept. Since everyone is subject to that reality, it helps me interact with people in an honest and compassionate way. To be a survivor, to me, means to feel in a deep sense both the wild capriciousness of life and the incredible wonder and mystery that exists in every moment.

Three or four years after moving to the West Coast, I decided I no longer wanted to fly back to Philly for my annual checkups. Deciding to move on to a new doctor felt like a significant transition and it was important for me to find a doctor who understood me and my history. I was beginning a new job and a new health plan and arrived at the initial visit with some nervousness. I told the doctor I had lymphoma and detailed the whole story. He began to do the checkup and, as he was feeling under my arm, he said, "I think I feel a lymph node. Definitely. I want to get you a test, an X ray and a blood test." It seemed as if he was almost excited to have an interesting case. I was devastated at the prospect of a relapse and angry at the idea that he may not have real expertise, and had acted presumptuously. I was on my way to work. When I left his office, I was trembling. I could not speak. I felt that he had little or no appreciation of what hearing his words might do to me.

I've grown to feel that, to some extent, everyone who is alive is a survivor. I don't feel nearly as distinguished from people who haven't had cancer as I might have before. I've realized that life has innate, built-in losses for everyone.

I went and sat in a park and I felt rage and astonishment at his callousness and felt that if indeed I had cancer, I would be tremendously crushed. It was a beautiful day and I wanted life so bad. I wanted simply to be able to see the blue sky and feel the wind. Two weeks later, I go back to this doctor to get the results of the tests. He doesn't even remember me! He had no memory of why he'd ordered the tests. He felt under my arm again and this time sensed nothing unusual. Nobody should be a doctor if he lacks the capacity to empathize.

The entire year after I finished school, I walked around with a fear of relapse. It spawned in me the realization of how much I loved life and really wanted to live. I think there can be a lot to gain from coming face-to-face with death and seeing that it is not something we have control over.

I'm glad to be thinking of these things because it makes me aware of the real truth of life. It has a lot to do with how I spend my time and what I do with myself. I don't believe that if I acquire material things it will make me happy. I'm not out to get rich or successful. I'm choosing to pay attention to people and act compassionately. This has rewards for me. My life would not have gone this way if I hadn't been sick. I could see myself trying hard to make a lot of money. I've chosen to become a teacher instead.

I would rather take life as both a blessing and a curse, rather than not have life. It's given me fortitude in difficult moments. To face the truth of my life meant that I was also going to

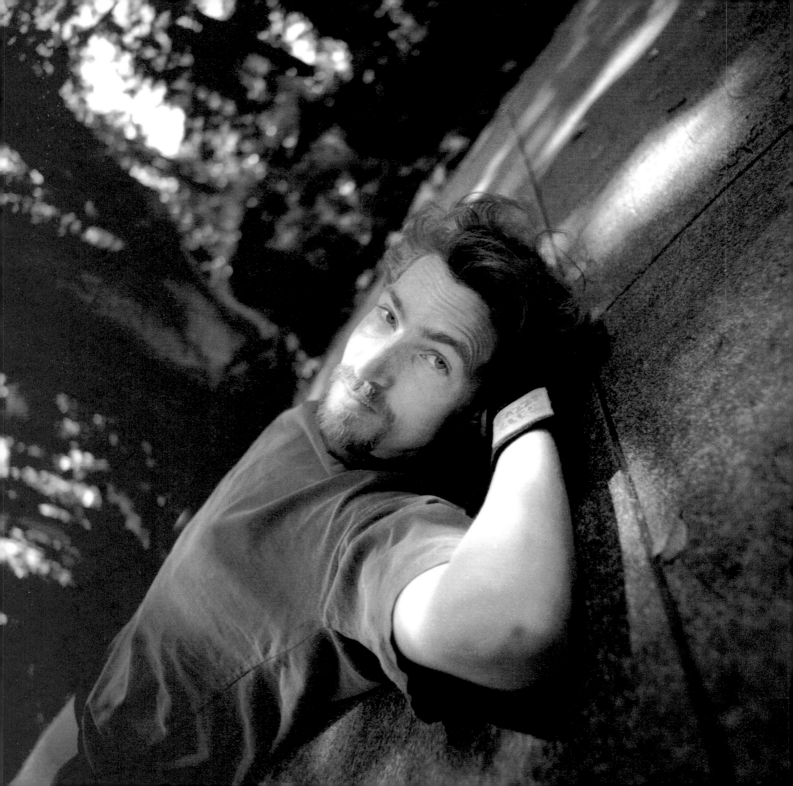

feel some pain. Well, when I had cancer, it made me more aware of how vulnerable I was. I know that tomorrow I could be in an emergency room being told that I have cancer or all kinds of things. If I knew that was going to happen to me in a month, how would I want to spend today? I would probably go to the YMCA and work out. I would enjoy the company of my friends or family. I would tell them I love them. I'd celebrate the people I'm with. This is not a thought I have every day. It comes and goes. But when it's with me, it's a benefit.

You only have this one life. You don't know what's left of it. There is going to be a last day. The worst thing for me would be to face that day and feel regretful. But there is nothing like recalling what it is like to be diagnosed, at the end of your rope, feeling beat-up, not having a choice or control. For me, there is no more powerful experience that has made it clear to me how to live my life. Now I make decisions that are more aligned with my heart. I'm on the path of no regret.

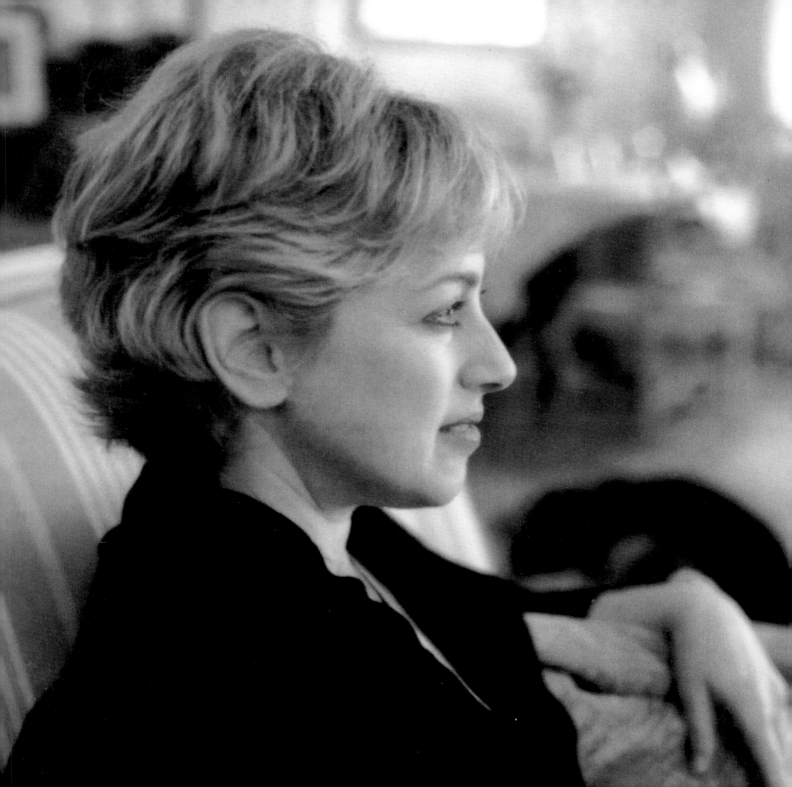

Susan Nessim

TWENTY-SIX-YEAR
SURVIVOR
RHABDOMYOSARCOMA

*A*T THE TIME I was diagnosed, I was at college in Boulder. I was seventeen. There was no patient empowerment then. The doctor was God, and you just did what he said. I was completely insolent and angry. I used to throw food at the doctors. I don't recommend that for everyone, but I think one reason I survived back then was that I wasn't one of those people who followed the rules.

College was really the first time I was ever away from my home in California. I was very superficial; just a sweet, lighthearted, carefree little girl—until I was diagnosed. That was the first thing that I knew had changed. Whatever my identity was before this disease, it was gone. I knew I was an outcast from my peer group and my family. It hit me that if I was going to fight, it was going to have to be from day one, or I was going to lose any part of myself that was recognizable.

I think that age is probably the hardest time to get cancer. You've just started to trust things in the world, people, yourself. And then that's taken away from you. I was a seventeen-year-old woman trying to come into her own. I was a virgin, going to college, trying to experience all these things. Then I am pulled back into the hospital—bald, eighty-five pounds, and fighting for my life.

It was the seventies and everyone was getting stoned and having sex, and I was stuck in the hospital puking. I thought, "If I'm going to die, I want to get laid!" But I think there is a sense that, when you have cancer and you have all this horrible treatment, you lose your desire to be loved or be held or have sex, because you're just this sick thing. By the time I got out of the hospital, I had very low self-esteem and I used the cancer card to keep people at a distance.

I remember going into a bank saying I wanted to start these support groups for survivors. The banker said, "You look great— what are you worried about? You got out of there; you got your hair back." I felt like smacking this man.

In my twenties I began to go to individual therapy. More important was my girlfriend Lisa, who I had met in the hospital. She was fifteen and had ovarian cancer. She and I were best friends. Cancervive was a selfish invention that Lisa and I started. Her health was deteriorating. She had lost the use of her legs and was in a wheelchair. She wanted to go down to Palm Springs, and I knew it was the last time we were going to spend together. I was so angry. She said, "We've got to do something about this—about us, survivors. Somebody should have told us that there were going to be long-term effects; that we were going to have trouble in the world after treatment." She came up with the name Cancervive for our organization.

The mission was to identify what survivorship issues were, and to help people prepare for when they walked out the hospital door. We wanted to give them a road map; some sort of safety net of therapy, information, and advice. We had our first support group in L.A., with

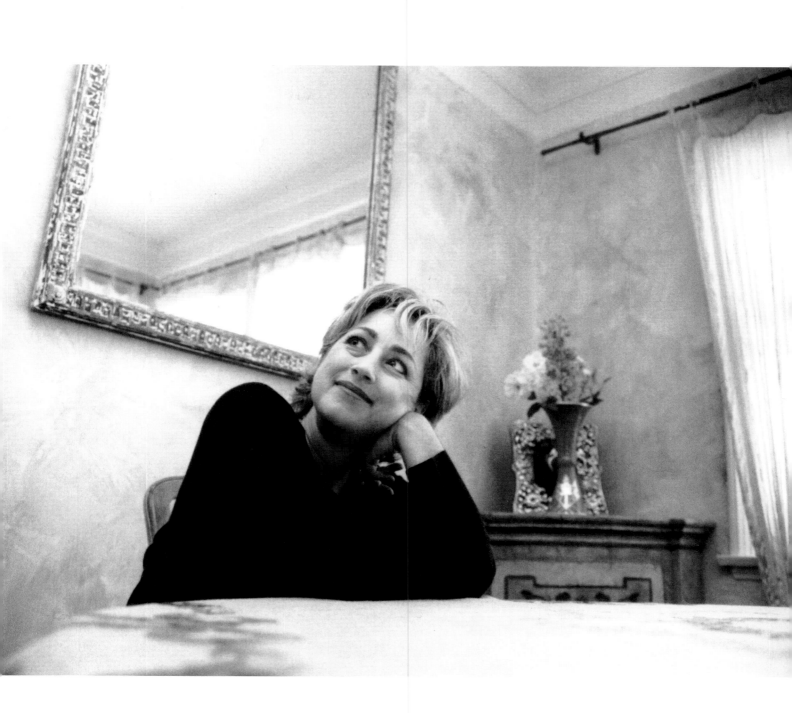

four other survivors. When Lisa died, I wanted to continue and see where it would take me. It's now been sixteen years.

I have a career around cancer, which has allowed me to do something positive with a horrible time in my life. It used to be that I couldn't be around other patients my age without getting depressed. Over time, I found that I could work through some of my own issues by seeing other people in a place where I had been, and realizing that I had come so far. There is a sort of exhilaration about being with people who are in a struggle for their life. It makes you remember what it was like for you, and to remember every day to live in a certain way. My husband says he's never known anyone but me who loves watching Holocaust films. I love the struggle; living on the edge. It's like always living each moment as if it's your last.

There's a part of me that doesn't want to associate the word cancer with myself anymore. There have been times when I just wanted to close Cancervive, shut the phones off. But then I just can't do it. I can't because I wouldn't want anyone to do it to me. I was dealing with my illness at a time when nobody reached out. I think there is so much value in it. No matter what a doctor tells you, if another survivor tells you something, you believe it.

I think discrimination against cancer patients and survivors is happening as much as it ever has. There's a kind of double-edged sword because cancer has come out of the closet. The health-insurance issue is never going to go away, and survivors still seem to take jobs that are less demanding because they don't want to be found out. That's sad to me, because I can't think of a stronger group or anyone I'd want to hire more.

It's much easier to get funding if you deal with patients, instead of survivorship. I remember going into a bank saying I wanted to start these support groups for survivors. The banker said, "You look great—what are you worried about? You got out of there; you got your hair back." I felt like smacking this man. That's the kind of attitude I've dealt with most of the time I've had Cancervive. What has changed is the separation of disease states. Because of the tremendous strides that have been taken with cancer, now there's the breast cancer movement, the prostate cancer movement, and so on. I find it a bit alarming. We are not all that different, but when you start splitting it off, I think it causes competition, politics, ugly stuff that doesn't need to be there.

I was still very angry about the way my body looked after treatment. I didn't walk around naked—everything was about covering up my body. My leg was swollen; I had a long, big scar on my thigh, and a limp. I got to the point where I thought, shit, I can't live like this. It was really stifling. Eventually, I started feeling stronger, more empowered from being around other people who knew what I was talking about. Little by little I started letting people in. It's only since I met my husband, Stephen, that I have felt comfortable letting anyone get really close to me. If a person didn't accept me, screw them. This is the leg, this is the package, and you've got your own package. Even so, it's only been in the last five years that I could look at myself as I was walking by a shop window.

I think the most important change for me, being a survivor, is the way I live. The way that I can reach other people. The relationships that I've made along the way—other survivors, people who didn't make it, my friend Lisa—and the things they taught me have sustained me. Recently I've felt so strong in my own skin; I know exactly who I am. I feel like I can do anything and be anything in this world. I've always felt I could walk into a situation and feel comfortable in it. That I can make friends wherever I am. That I can be taken seriously. People sense that I'm not someone to be trifled with. I will stand up for people and for what I believe. I don't know many people like that. I think it's because I'm a survivor.

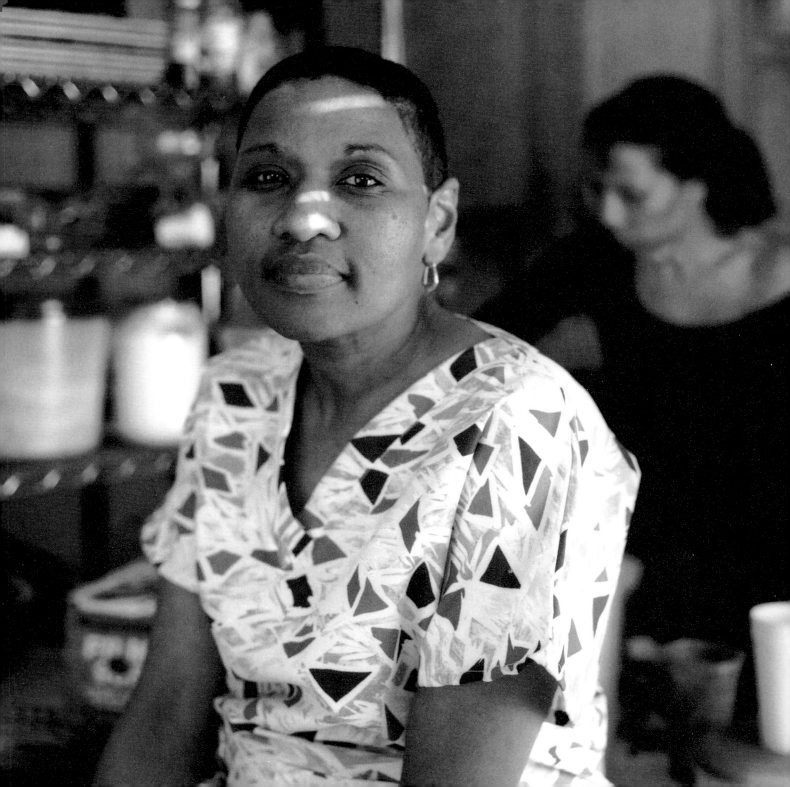

Cynthia Pitre

SEVEN-YEAR SURVIVOR
BREAST CANCER

*I*WAS DIAGNOSED IN February 1994, eleven days after my thirty-seventh birthday. When I first heard the news I just thought. "What is this about, God?" I didn't feel fear immediately. In my church we study that disease is part of emotional and spiritual imbalance, so I started hunting for answers to where my imbalance lay.

I kept calm. I told just a few friends because I didn't want to get into their fears of death, or be afraid of the diagnosis. I only told friends who were highly spiritual and who could affirm my healing.

I had a lumpectomy but they did not get a clear margin. About two weeks later we did another mammogram and sonogram and, lo and behold, the cancer had spread and my breast kept getting harder and harder. This was when I really started feeling the fear. I went for several other opinions and the doctors all wanted to do more surgery, maybe with chemo or radiation. But that just wasn't what I wanted to hear.

One day I went to the health food store in between doctor's appointments and I found this thin book called *Beating Cancer with Nutrition*. I sat on that floor and I read that book with tears in my eyes. I felt like this was maybe something I could do besides take the breast off.

I found a doctor who had healed herself from liver cancer forty-one years ago in a similar way. She said, "I want you to clear out every animal flesh, every dairy product in your house, every canned good, every processed food, every box. And I want you to fill it up with raw vegetables and raw fruit. I want you to drink sixty-four ounces of carrot juice with a lot of green raw vegetables every day. And I want you to have a gallon of water a day, and don't you forget that gallon of water, because it's important. Every Friday I want you to come in here for at least five and a half months to do colon irrigation." I didn't even ask her what that meant.

At thirty-two, I had arthritis. At thirty-four, I was feeling old age. As I moved higher up in the executive world, my stress level got bigger and, because I was running away from the fear of poverty, I worked my butt off. I had lots of friends and I did a lot of different things. But my whole life changed when I had breast cancer. The total focus became enhancing my spiritual world, healing myself emotionally and physically.

It was very difficult at first to eat only raw vegetables and fruit. I dreamed of meat and of all the foods I loved to eat. During the healing crisis, while my body detoxed, I was very tired and run-down. It felt like I had the flu. My nose was running all the time, my eyes were watering, my ears were very waxy, and there were times when I could not hold my head up. I would drink my carrot juice and I would sleep like I hadn't slept in years.

Over time, I noticed physical changes. I watched my eyes and skin clearing up and brightening. And I would touch my hair and it was so soft. By the eighth week all my allergies were gone and I've never had a breathing problem since. I was jumping for joy. I knew this breast cancer was going to be going, if it already wasn't gone

By the eighth or ninth week of the new diet, the pain in the breast had gone away; I couldn't feel the lump anymore by the third and fourth month. So six months and nine days later, I did my mammogram. The nurse came back and looked at me and said, "The doctor can see nothing but benign tissue." I hugged her and said, "I told you." And I went out of the hospital hugging everybody—people I didn't even know. The doctor called me and said, "Congratulations, you're a medical miracle." They did six-month checkups all the way up to three years and finally they put it in writing: "No evidence of cancer."

But I was preaching to the world. I told my friends to do colon irrigation, change their diet, start juicing. I opened up my center to do colon irrigation and nutritional counseling out of my house. It was unbelievable how fast it grew through word of mouth. And I got into it with all my heart. I continued to grow spiritually and tried my best to bring that light into people, but I realized that they needed to find their own emotional healing. They had to do the work, and it took a lot of discipline. It's not easy going this route. I was mad for a while at doctors because they don't come out more often to explain the alternatives.

In the beginning, I had my challenges. I stayed away from my friends' houses. I didn't get caught in restaurants. If friends came over, they knew to bring something raw. After five and a half months I was able to do cooked foods, but still strictly vegan. I learned how to make vegetarian foods that would satisfy everybody else, so I was back into socializing more often, but I had lost a lot of friends. You lose the environment that you're so used to, because food is a social thing. You go on a date, and he brings you to eat, right? Guess what—your whole lifestyle is going to change. It did for me. But you wouldn't believe how many of my friends have converted. Today, cancer doesn't scare me.

The survivor and the victor—sometimes they overlap. I'm cured. I'm a victor. The difference is that I made a drastic change and make sure that every part of my life is around my health. Every single minute. Most people do not wake up in the morning and say, "What do

One day I went to the health food store in between doctor's appointments and I found this thin book called Beating Cancer with Nutrition. *I sat on that floor and I read that book with tears in my eyes. I felt like this was maybe something I could do besides take the breast off.*

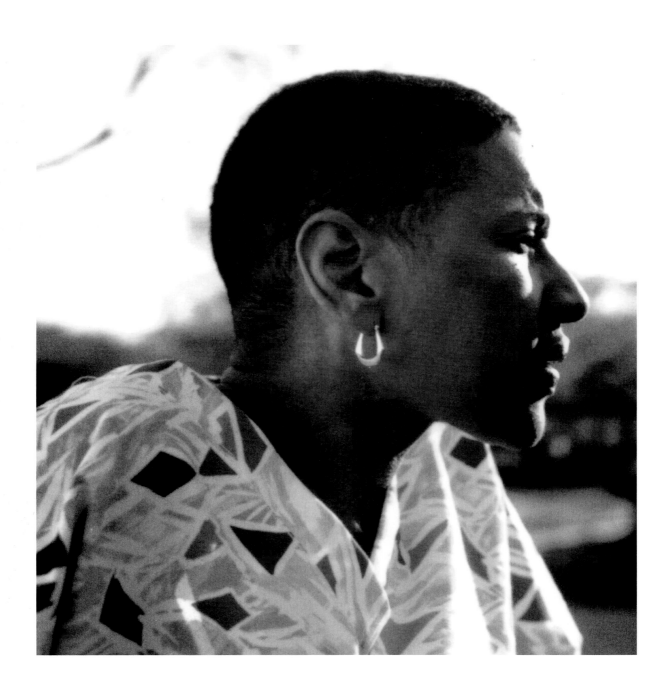

I need to put in my body that's healthy, that's going to get me through the day? Where am I going to go to get it? What time? Will I be available to get that item to live for the day?" Instead, we wake up and think, "Got to drop off the kids, got to get to work, call this person, be there from eight to five, and maybe in between I'll go over here and get something quick to eat." A disease cannot grow in a true, healthy body the way God made it. I've reversed everything that was going on with my body.

To handle stress, I do a massage every week. I work out four to five times a week. I meditate. And when there are emotions I let myself emote. There is still some imbalance in that area because God has taken me so fast on the growth of my business. Now my center is in a 2,800-square-foot house. I've got ten employees, an herbalist, a lady who does food preparation, and a naturopath doctor. People are calling left and right. My cup runneth over. And I'm one person who's trying to delegate. I want more time to get real quiet.

I'm a visionary. One day I want to have a hospital. God says, "I want you to do more things here. I will provide everything you need." And I'm going, "God, You're not doing it fast enough!"

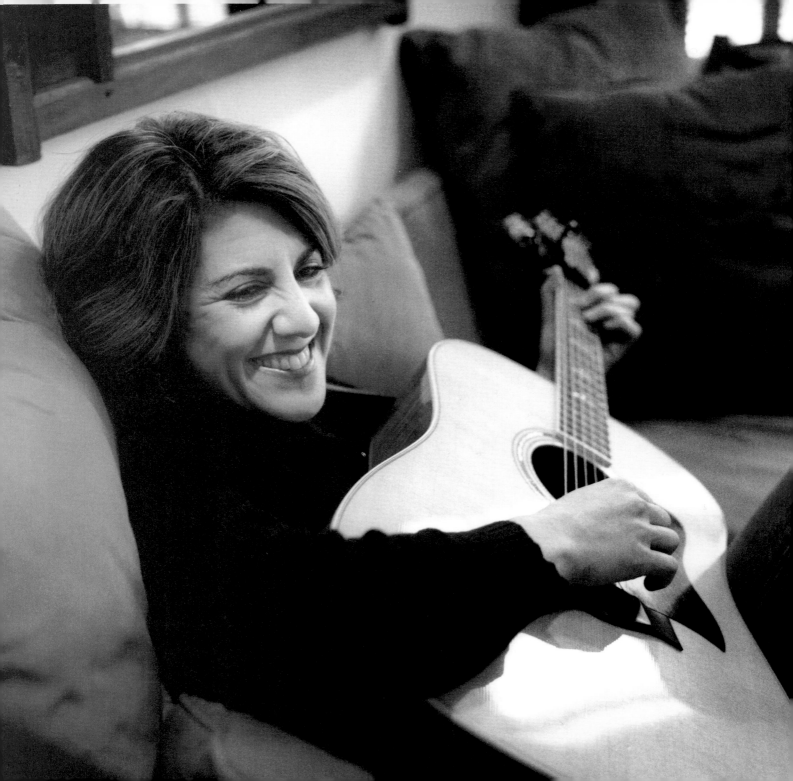

Peri Smilow

TWO-YEAR SURVIVOR
CERVICAL CANCER

■

I WAS DIAGNOSED with cervical cancer in January 2000. I didn't have any obvious symptoms except unusual bleeding and an abnormal Pap smear, until they did a D & C, gathering cells from my cervix and uterus to biopsy. From the second I got the diagnosis, my total mode of operation was to take charge and gather information: "Okay, spell 'squamous cell' for me. Tell me what that means." I asked a lot of questions. The only piece of information I didn't want to hear was survival statistics. I decided I didn't give a fuck—I am a statistic of one. I got off the phone with the doctor and thought, "Life as I know it has just changed."

I always knew I had really deep faith, but I had no idea how deep it was. I was incredibly strong for the first month. I put my head down and just went through it. It's taken two years for me to give myself permission to be angry. But all the way through, my general feeling was that I had to put very good karma out in the world.

I was prepared to have a hysterectomy if that was going to save my life. But as soon as I learned that I had to have one, I felt like it was like a trade with the devil: "Here's the deal. I give you my uterus, I get to live. How's that?"

Bud and I had only been dating about four months before the diagnosis, but we had already started talking about getting married and having children. I thought I was a pretty sophisticated person in the world. I always thought that you could harvest eggs the way they harvest sperm, but you can't. It turns out that it takes several menstrual cycles, and they have to be impregnated before you can store them. Given that fact, and that I didn't want our relationship decided by the fact that we had these eggs sitting in a cooler someplace, we didn't do it. I had always thought I would adopt a child, so I wasn't far away from that concept. But it still continues to be an issue in our relationship, and we talk about it a lot.

Part of what kept me going during those early weeks was that we had to either dance or laugh every day. Bud brought a couple of CDs of massive Motown, and we would dance to Aretha. If it wasn't Aretha, we were listening to Bill Cosby, or Mel Brooks's *The 2000 Year Old Man*, laughing hysterically.

Now, I have a very hard struggle around my anniversaries. I knew that if there was going to be a recurrence of cervical cancer, it's most likely to occur in the first two years. So, for two years I said to myself, gotta make it to two. Bud asked me to marry him but I couldn't then. I wasn't ready.

This weekend I am moving to New York City to be with Bud. And we're planning our wedding. I think I am willing to make the move now because I was sick. No one is writing me any promises about anything. I damn well better move on and take risks. How long can I dig my heels in and say I want to have a partner, and still not go? Trying out a new mode for myself is not comfortable, but I think, "Well, I never had cancer before either." I made it through that, so let's go. Take it on.

I'm struggling to maintain the pre-cancer me and to stay in touch with who was I before. There've been a lot of times that I wanted to go back to my old touchstones. I'd want to go back to my old job, relationships, stuff that was familiar. I can't. That's gone. That's been very hard for me because I still have a lot of processing to do around my cancer. I think about it a lot. I am very proud of how I got through cancer, but now I want things to be easy. I want to pamper myself. I just want to revel in the "Woe is me" a little bit, which is not my personality. Then I say to myself, "What are you talking about, girlfriend? Get over that!"

I went through a period of time where I was afraid to go out after my surgery. I felt like I was wearing a "C"—that everyone was going to know I had cancer, and I didn't want them to know. At a certain point, that flipped. I realized that I'm different than I used to be. Now I *need* people to know. Because if they don't know I had cancer, how will they know that I'm different?

I've had a deep, deep need to create a legacy. If I couldn't have children, then I wanted to leave a body of work that would be me. As an artist and musician, I have been exploring that whole idea of legacy and what that is for me. I express myself through music, but I haven't written a single song since I got sick. It's taken a long time for me to want to use my art to talk about it.

I was prepared to have a hysterectomy if that was going to save my life. But as soon as I learned that I had to have one, I felt like it was like a trade with the devil: "Here's the deal. I give you my uterus, I get to live. How's that?"

I spend my professional life now as a public person. In the last few years my career has gone national. It's in the Jewish music world, so it's a small world, but in that small world I am becoming famous. I'm aware that this gives me a pulpit to do things and say things. I learned that when people know I had cancer, they become more receptive. There is this sense that what I say has more weight somehow.

My life's work, before I got sick and after, is about leaving the planet a better place than when I came, and trying to get others to do the same. I'm realizing that having had cancer is actually a wonderful tool if I can use it well, and not abuse it. It's like an energy running alongside me. If I can find a way to not resent or hate it, not be scared by it, then it will make the rest of my life's work that much more powerful.

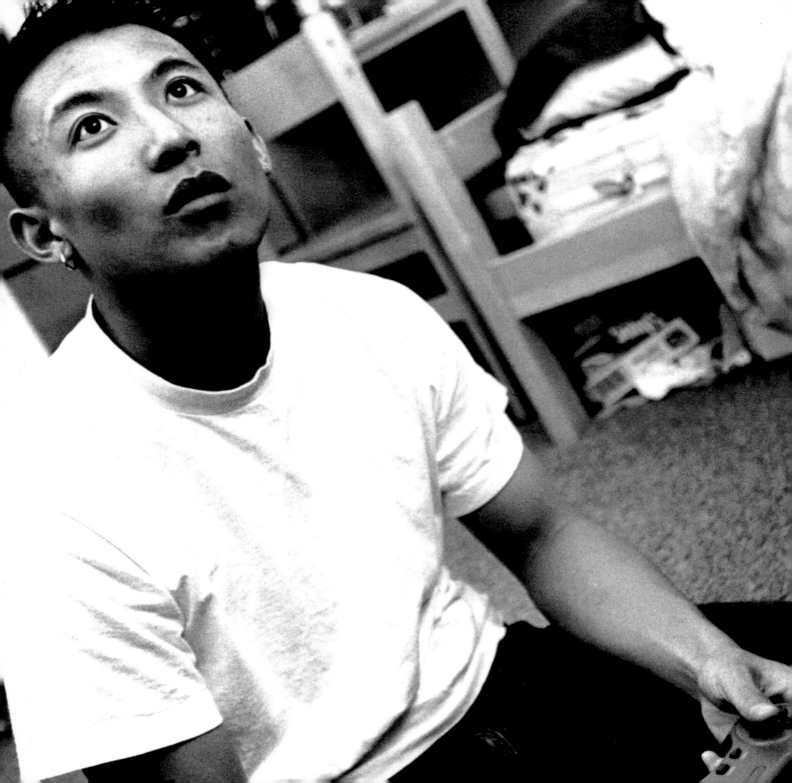

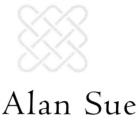

Alan Sue

TWO-YEAR SURVIVOR
OSTEOGENIC SARCOMA

WHEN I WAS sixteen, this guy pulled a gun on the street and shot at my head. Some of my friends and I beat him up. During the fight, I lost my balance. I fell and my leg broke just above my knee, in the thigh bone. The bone had been really brittle because a tumor was there, but I didn't know that at the time.

My parents told me I had cancer but I just went back to sleep. After that, I was in and out of the hospital for a year. I thought I was going to die but I didn't really care. I had so many things going on in my life. I'd just broken up with my girlfriend and was depressed. I didn't like where I was living. I didn't see my parents too often 'cause I was out most of the time and it didn't seem like they really cared.

After I got sick my relationship with them got better. We moved and they seemed to try to make life better for me and my sister. I never really talked to them. My dad's not a real emotional guy and my mom doesn't speak English. We can't express much to each other. I was crying a lot. It seemed like it was just me and my sister.

I grew up in the ghetto and there were a lot of gang guys around me. I was way involved with them. It was like the jungle. I didn't even know the guy who pulled the gun. He walked by and elbowed me in the stomach so I figured he was a bad guy. After I got sick, I didn't change the people I was hanging around with. They were there for me. They stuck by me.

I can still feel my toes. I can move my knee and foot and toes and ankle in my head. When I get the phantom pain, I think it's the devil wanting me to join him. It's like I'm being tugged down.

When they told me I was going to lose my leg, I thought it might be kind of cool. I was just so glad to be rid of the cancer. But after it was gone, I regretted it. Then I started to miss it. I started to ask, "Why?" and "How?" and blamed things on the cancer. I started blaming my mom for her cooking and all kinds of things. I always blame that guy who made me fall.

I took chemo for a year even though they took my leg. They didn't cut all of it off; they wanted to save my hip even though there was some cancer there. When I started trying to date again I got rejected a lot. I was self-conscious even though I was ready to show people who I really am. I stayed low, didn't do much. I was afraid to do things because I didn't want to look stupid. I began to wear baggier clothes to make my leg look less fake.

Now, I've started going dancing again. I thought that I should be more outgoing, do more that usually made me afraid, like bowling. I always thought I had to have a running start, but now I just go up and throw the ball. A couple of times I knocked all the balls down.

When I see amputees outside, I don't look at them funny or think twice. I'm just paranoid about myself. It's a big change and I get afraid of rejection. The little kids make fun of how I walk. They limp when they see me. I feel bad for a second, but then I tell myself that it's okay, they're just kids and they don't know any better.

Last year my dad talked to me, saying I was the last kid and I should go to a good college. I applied to all the UC schools and Santa Cruz accepted me. My parents were really excited about me getting in but they were afraid because it was far from San Francisco. They got me a car so I could get home on the weekends. I'm not expected to go home, but they like me to and that's where all my friends are. When I go home, we shoot pool or eat, or go to karaoke, or race on the freeway at night.

Believe it or not, having cancer has made me less of a daredevil. It's made me appreciate what I have more. I look for better ways of fulfilling my wishes.

I kind of just go with the flow now. I don't really think a lot about my cancer coming back, but it's in my head. I just want to be happy. I'm seeing someone now who I really like. She's strong and smart and beautiful. She thinks the world of me. She wants me to go swimming one day, but I'm too shy right now. I won't have my leg and the kids will all say, "Ha, ha, ha, look at that boy! How come he doesn't have a leg?"

Her friends like me, too, and I thought they might be kind of sick of me 'cause I'm a burden. When I'm with them they can't do physical stuff. But they say it doesn't matter; it's okay. I'm trying to be more outgoing for her, but I don't know if I'll ever be totally unselfconscious.

I never thought about what I wanted to do when I got older. I do now. Before, I looked for someone to take my anger out on. Now I just punch walls. During cancer I had a lot of holes in my walls. There was something happening to me that I couldn't do anything about. I felt out of control. I didn't feel like I was in the right body, but I just had to tell myself to stay calm. I talked my way through things. I saw a shrink. I talked about my dreams. I had a lot of guns in my dreams.

My doctors tried to get me to go to groups and to talk to other kids about what I'd been through. I didn't go. I tried to do everything *but* think about cancer. But I can't escape it—I have to put my leg on every morning.

I have bad memories of the phantom pain. That's real. It feels like needles, like when your arm falls asleep, with a little bit of pain too. It lasted all day and all night. I had it for about six months before it got better. Now it's better, but I get weird twitches. I can still feel my toes. I can move my knee and foot and toes and ankle in my head. When I get the phantom pain, I think it's the devil wanting me to join him. It's like I'm being tugged down.

This summer I had to go to a special class here, at school. I had a roommate and for the first three weeks I didn't tell him; I would just take off my leg under my blanket. After that, I decided to tell Larry, my roommate now, the very first day of school. He just accepted it from the first day. He's been great about it. He doesn't care if I take my leg off in the room, but I still go in the bathroom.

I think I've come a long way. I've stayed away from gangs and started concentrating more on school and drawing. Drawing was just a gift I was born with. I remember drawing as a really little kid. For me, it's all about fantasy and being able to create whatever I want. I can draw a big buff man and a little guy. Versions of me.

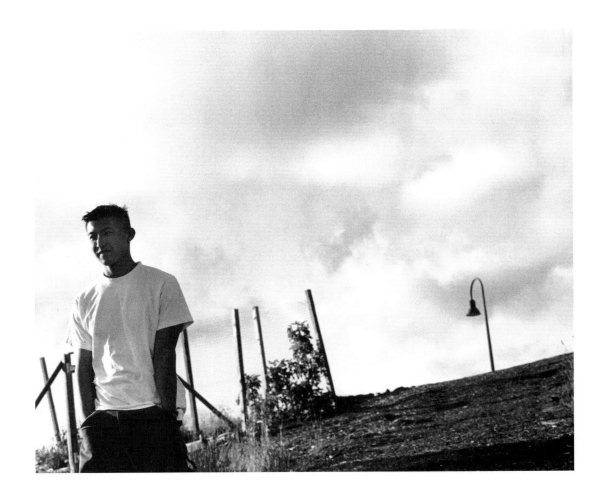

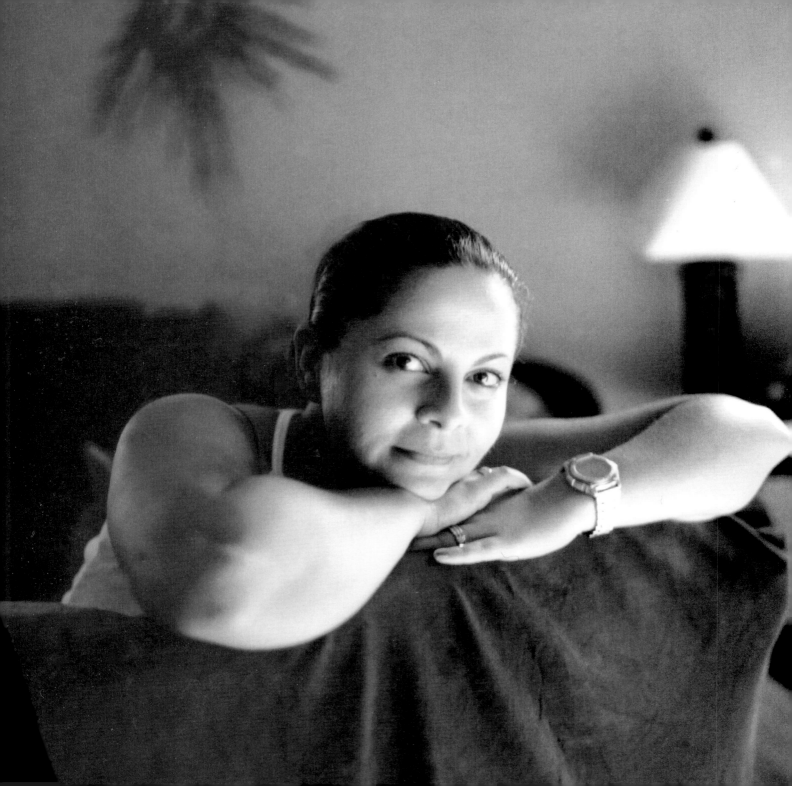

Fairuz Benyousef

FOURTEEN-YEAR SURVIVOR
HODGKIN'S DISEASE

*E*VEN THOUGH MY father had gone through leukemia and was in remission, I just couldn't fathom that something like cancer would ever happen to me.

The first time we came to the United States from Libya was in 1973. We stayed for four years while my parents got their degrees, then we went back to Libya. We came back to Harrisburg in 1980, when I was eight, for my mom and dad to pursue their doctorate degrees at Penn State. Within a couple of years, my dad was diagnosed with leukemia. In Libya, cancer was one of the worst things you could ever be afflicted with.

When we started to put this all in perspective, we started asking whether it had something to do with the 1979 accident at Three Mile Island, because there was no other history in the family of cancer. It wasn't very far away from where we lived and the incidence of cancer was very high. Everyone you talked to, somebody was getting some kind of cancer.

I don't remember a whole lot about my father's treatment, although it lasted a couple of years. He ended up being in remission about a year before I was diagnosed with Hodgkin's. I was about to go into tenth grade and I was on top of the world.

I remember very clearly the look on my father's face the day I had to have bone marrow withdrawn. It was comforting that he knew what I was going through, but it was also horrible because my dad was such a sensitive man that I could see it, in turn, paining him. It was never a spoken thing, but it reassured me that I knew we could relate on this level.

I tried to protect him at times. I think I tried to walk in his footsteps. I saw how strong he was when he went through his first leukemia, and I wanted to be strong like he was. I had been cancer-free for about a year and a half when he relapsed. It was a very short and aggressive kind of attack, and a bone marrow transplant didn't work.

Unlike most moms and teenage daughters who tend to separate, my mother and I fused even more because of the cancer experience. Mom had lost a husband, she had a daughter who had a serious illness, I had lost a father whom I was very close to—she was stuck to me and I was stuck to her.

In Middle Eastern and Islamic societies, the family is extremely important and the core of the social system. Mom was a Ph.D. but, in her world, girls don't go to college and live on campus because there are boys around, and what if someone tries to make the moves on you? Between the illnesses and being displaced culturally, we had a lot of issues about separating.

At the end of this year I'm going to turn thirty and, more than ever before, I've been thinking about what it means to have gone through what I did—maybe because I'm more settled and thinking about starting a family. I still think terrible thoughts. Are my children going to have a greater chance of disease because of what's happened to me and my father? I hope to God they get the stamina and health genes from my husband, who's a soccer coach, because I think it's even more difficult for a loved one to witness the pain of a disease. I do not want to one day be in my mother's shoes, watching what happened to me happen to my kids.

The good thing about all this, though, is being a lot more aware of the body that I do have. I try to take good care of myself—more than some of my friends who are the same age—and if I do start to feel ill, not wait to do something about it. I'm diligent about going annually to get my checkups; I take the initiative with the doctor to ask questions and to probe issues about whatever I might have read or heard, or whatever they say to me that doesn't make sense.

My mom is a food scientist and nutritionist, so she started me on an intensive regimen of supplements. I'm not always religious about it, but even if I go off for a week or two, I always come back. That, exercise, trying to have a healthy diet, just the normal stuff, but also looking— I'm always looking at my collarbone and my lymph nodes. I don't know if it's control or just needing to be aware, because the doctors of course put the fear of God into you about it coming back.

My dad's illness and mine have definitely shaped how I approach all relationships with people close to me. Maybe most is the issue of never thinking, "Oh, these people will always be there." For a long time, I couldn't understand why, if my husband went away on a soccer trip, I'd get so emotional about it, crying and crying. Finally it hit me that here was another very close man in my life, and the issue of loss was just hovering all over me; I was fearing that I'd never see him again. It was very, very difficult to let go of that. It's still tough that he has to go away, but I think just discovering what it was, putting my finger on it, has helped me.

Prayer was very important when I was sick. I remember my mom and dad saying Dua'aa, a prayer that everything would work out, have a long healthy life, that kind of thing. I remember my dad, even when he was at his sickest, still maintaining his prayers. The wonderful thing about Islam is that it's a religion of ease if you're sick or unable. Even if you're immobile and on your back, you can pray with your eyes. You can actually do the motion of the kneeling and the coming up and, in your heart, just be saying a prayer.

Unlike most moms and teenage daughters who tend to separate, my mother and I fused even more because of the cancer experience. Mom had lost a husband, she had a daughter who had a serious illness, I had lost a father whom I was very close to—she was stuck to me and I was stuck to her.

I relied heavily on my faith in God and belief in Islam that this world we're in right now is temporary; that the hereafter is truly what it's all about, instead of just holding on to life here. You know, whatever is meant to be is meant to be. I mean, I'm not going to sit on my butt and not get treatment, or just wait and say, "Oh God, whatever You want is fine," because I don't think that's right. But faith was very important and just believing that things do happen for a reason.

I've been told that people who don't know me very well think of me as, not stuck-up, but a career woman. Somebody who's got it together, someone who's not tough, but certainly serious, organized. As I get to know them, telling them I had cancer perhaps humbles me to them, makes me more real and less of a Superwoman.

The funny thing about the cancer is, sure it's a victory and I'm a survivor, thank goodness, but I don't see it like a Superwoman—like, "I did it." It's not fundamentally *me* that made that happen. It goes back to my faith and God, and things happening that are not in my control.

As a woman, outside the issues with the cancer, our society is not very forgiving to begin with. So many of my girlfriends are always worried about their stomach this and their stomach that. I have learned to love my muscles and my curves and I don't ever want to have a flat belly. It's a struggle, but I'm just happy to have a body that's healthy. I've got this beautiful scar right above my belly button where my spleen was removed and I love it, I really do. It's a great reminder of what I went through. Of my victory.

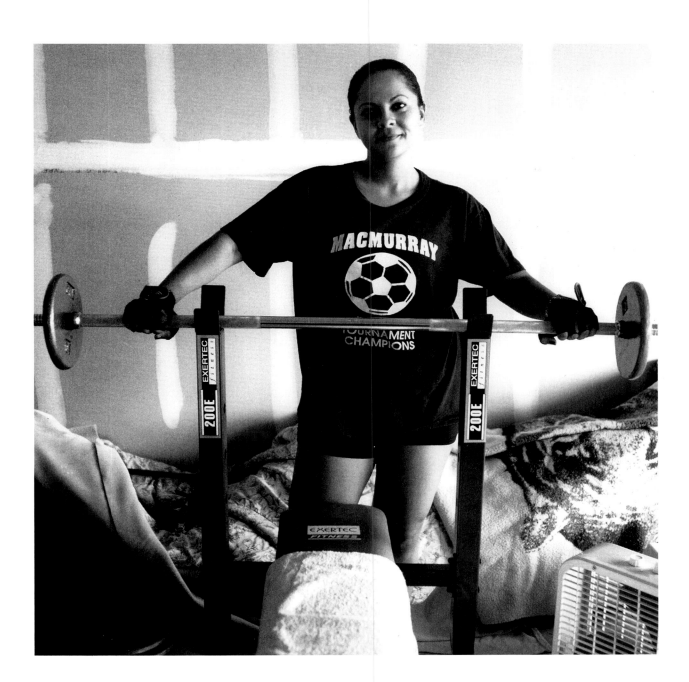

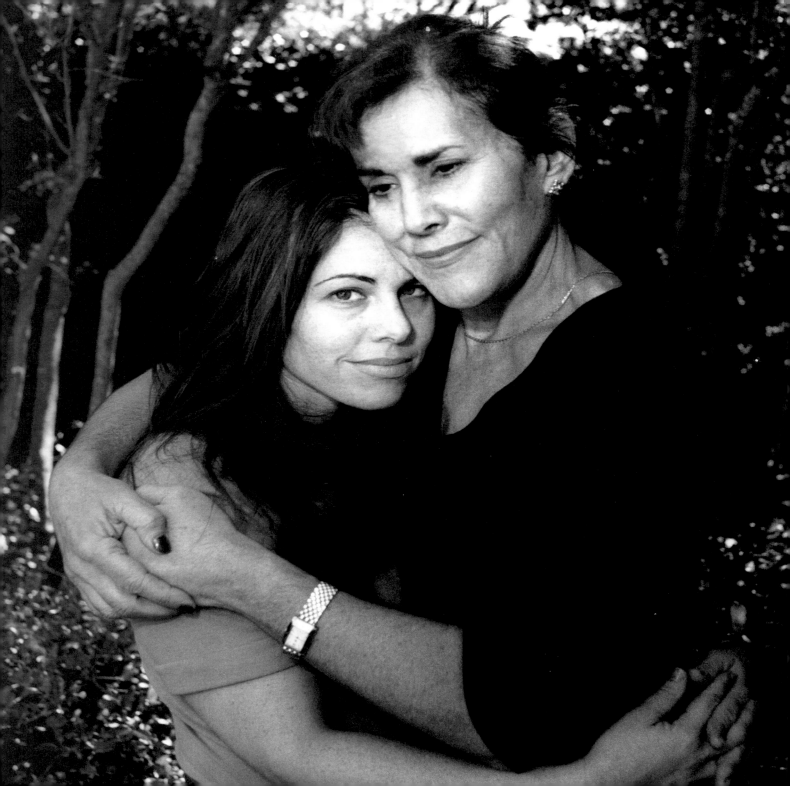

Nikki Jeffords

SIX-YEAR SURVIVOR
BREAST CANCER

■

WHEN I WAS thirty-seven I had a waking dream that told me I had breast cancer. Just like that. I decided to get myself checked out, in case. I had always had this need to have mammograms, even thought it wasn't recommended for women my age, with no history of cancer. But, I wanted to have a baseline. I always went with my sister because it freaked me out.

I was told I was fine, but I still felt tense. Just after, I had a dream of my father, who had died ten years before. This

NIKKI JEFFORDS WITH HER DAUGHTER JOFKA

dream was unlike any other that I'd had because he was so real. I walked up and put my arms around him. I was so happy to see him. I looked at his face and it was extremely sad and then it faded away.

The following week, I got a call that they had found something in my breast and it was very clear it was not just a cyst. At first, I thought I was going to lose my breast and that was pretty horrific. Then I thought I was going to lose my hair, and then I thought I was probably going to die.

I had been told to picture the tumor and surround it with white light. I hated doing that.

I'd had problems with severe anxiety. I was always worrying, about my kids, my work, the tiny little things I had to do. I had also been in AA for about thirteen years. I used the program philosophy, "One day at a time," more for my cancer than when I was getting sober.

Initially, I had a lumpectomy but there were complications. They ultimately had to go back in and they found the tumor in the duct, which is good in terms of it not spreading, but bad in terms of recurrence. They thought I was better off just getting rid of the whole breast.

My biggest fear was for my kids. My oldest was twenty-five, my middle nine, and my youngest four. I thought that I couldn't leave them or my husband, George, because they were not ready for me to go. I remembered when George and I met and it just made me weep. I kept telling him that if anything should go wrong, he should remarry.

I went through my negative reactions very quickly and then had the feeling that I had to see things positively. I had been told to picture the tumor and surround it with white light. I hated doing that. I read a lot of books on breast cancer and they made me really depressed. If I had to give advice to anyone, it would be to do whatever feels right for *you*. If that means sitting around eating ice cream and sobbing, go that route. Don't do anything that feels like pulling teeth. Once I gave up doing that stuff, I felt better.

Now there is so much more information. At the time, I didn't even know what reconstruction looked like. So I went and started looking for reconstructed breasts. I went to see three women, and every breast looked different. At least I knew I was going to be able to have a breast, and that was reassuring. Now, anyone who wants to see my breasts absolutely can. You really can't even tell, they're done so fantastically well these days.

I went into menopause the second month I was on chemo. I lost my libido entirely. It was like losing a limb. I didn't realize how much tamoxifen killed my sex drive until I went off it. This wasn't good for my marriage. We became like two ships passing in the night. I was kind of stupid about that because I really thought that ignoring my husband was all right. Within twenty-four hours of going off the tamoxifen, I felt different. I felt more buoyant. I started feeling normal again, alive down there. I began to court my husband and we're having sex all the time now. I'm in my second adolescence!

Two or three years after my first mastectomy, I got a questionnaire in the mail asking about how depressed and terrible did I feel having breast cancer? I couldn't believe it, because I was feeling great. I had made changes that were positive. I bought a horse to ride with my daughter; I got someone to help me clean the house. We moved and I wrote a novel that was going to be published. I gave myself time to enjoy stuff, and laughter became more important. I found a new direction with my work and, since, have been feeling really productive.

A few months ago, I had my other breast removed. I decided to have a preventative mastectomy because my breast surgeon recommended it strongly, in view of the fact that I was off tamoxifen and had started taking a form of estrogen called estriol. I felt much better taking estriol—sexier, more feminine, calmer, softer. The breast surgeon was not convinced the hormone was okay for the breast and said I was caught between two schools of thought. Basically, it was either be happy and get rid of the breast, or get off hormones. I opted for happy.

I made the decision within a week of having seen the breast surgeon, and I made it without qualms. By then I'd realized how high the statistics were of recurrence in the other breast. I didn't want to take the chance. The fact that my insurance was going to pay helped make up my mind. Also, I had a good plastic surgeon and knew I'd be perfectly happy with a reconstructed breast. My family and friends were supportive. The surgery was a bit of an ordeal, although reconstruction from the stomach seems easier than from the back. If I could do it all over again, I'd have both breasts removed the first time around. I would advise most women do the same until they come up with a better solution.

It took a full six weeks to recover, but now I feel great, have lost a lot of the extra weight I put on with the hormones, and feel good about my body image. They did find some atypical cells, so I know I did the right thing, but I will always worry about cancer. Though I certainly feel more relaxed than I was before, I'll always be scared of it showing up in my body again.

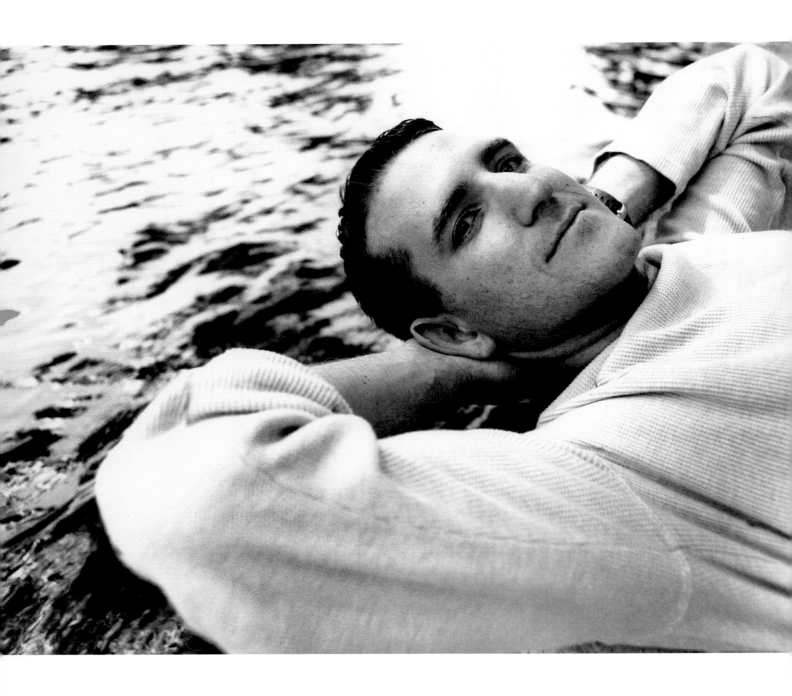

Doug Ulman

FIVE-YEAR SURVIVOR
CHONDROSARCOMA,
MELANOMA

I WAS GETTING ready to start my sophomore year in college when I found out I had cancer—chondrosarcoma—which usually occurs in cartilage. Not exactly a household word, and definitely something I had never heard of. I had a major chest resection and they took out part of my rib cage with the tumors.

There was a lot of discussion as to whether I should have further treatment and we went to specialist after specialist. That's probably as helpless as I have ever felt, but I kept pushing. My parents taught me not to just accept the first answer that you get, and to stand up for who you are and what you believe in. I can totally sympathize that this is difficult for a lot of people, but I think that an experience like cancer teaches you that you either do it or you don't. And if you don't, then you are leaving yourself in the hands of the system, which may or may not be beneficial.

I was nineteen, majoring in American history and education at Brown University and playing varsity soccer. We were going into that season ranked seventh in the country. I was probably in the best shape of my life. Kind of a cliché—life is good, then cancer.

When I went back to school after the surgery, my soccer coach called a team meeting, and that's when I told everybody what was going on. I encouraged everybody on the team to ask questions; don't be afraid to talk about it. That was probably one of the hardest things I had to do. I looked around the room and realized that, including myself, nobody here had dealt with this. Nobody knew how to react. Some people came up and gave me a hug and other people kind of steered away because they just weren't sure what to do. I sat in the locker room after everybody had gone out to practice and just cried.

My coach taught me that if you don't set a goal, you won't achieve what you really want. We set a goal that I would suit up and play by the end of the season. He had already outfitted my whole locker with all the practice gear and stuff, so I'd put it on and sit there and watch practice. After six weeks I could play again, and I probably played the best soccer of my life. I wanted to play so bad. I told my good friends and my parents I was going to play in a game, and they all came into town. I played about fifty-five minutes and we won. And that was the end of my season. I mean, I woke up the next day and I couldn't walk. But I still went to all the games and practiced.

Around that time, I saw a *PrimeTime Live* special that Sam Donaldson and Judd Rose did about their own cancers. They talked about how we've come so far in cancer but we have so far to go, and we really need people to get involved and do things in the cancer world. I called my mom that night and said, "Look, we gotta do something." Because I was playing soccer, the story had gotten some publicity, and I thought we could raise money. I didn't know what it would turn into, but I thought we might as well try to raise some money to give to somebody to start programs for young adults. So that's how we started the Ulman Cancer Fund.

In March and June of that same school year I was diagnosed with melanoma. The first time, they took out this big chunk of tissue, did some tests and said it was melanoma in situ, encapsulated. You're fine. Go back to school. I had no idea at that point how dangerous it was or that I'd probably have another.

When I went to see my dermatologist for my next checkup, they removed another mole. It came back invasive melanoma and I had surgery three weeks later. I had learned that melanoma is actually the most prevalent cancer in people in their twenties—another cancer that affects young adults, and one that's preventable. It reinforced the need for talking with somebody who had been through this, so getting the fund up and running became more important to me.

Today, the Ulman Fund provides young adult support groups in five cities. They're mostly geared toward people in their twenties and thirties. They're all professionally facilitated; they're all free. For the most part, they're unstructured, just a place to talk, and there's a social aspect. We also match people up over email. We offer scholarships to people pursuing higher education—grad school, undergrad, trade school—who have had cancer and can't afford school.

I think, in general, I'm kind of an entrepreneur. I always like doing and starting new things. If the Ulman Cancer Fund does nothing for the next fifty years, every time we hear the National Cancer Institute or American Cancer Society or the large cancer centers really taking young adult issues seriously, we know we helped get people to start addressing it, which I think is awesome.

Leaving the Ulman Fund to come work at the Lance Armstrong Foundation was a very hard decision. Lance knew what I had done and I think he saw that, with a budget of $150–200,000 a year, I had done a lot. It's hard to leave something that you've started, but I needed to do what was best for my own personal development. I was finally okay with leaving because the Ulman Fund was financially stable, with money in the bank and an endowment.

It's easier to get away from the work than it is from the cancer. The cancer, it's always, "Where's the sunscreen, where's your wide-brimmed hat?" None of my friends are doing that. When I go play golf, usually I wear long pants. There's always a constant reminder. But on the flip side, I'm the only one that's happy when it's cloudy and rainy.

It's hard for me to turn work off, because I don't see what I do as my "job." My personal mission is to help as many people as possible. It's like a calling. Sometimes I think that's hard for my girlfriend, Dana, to understand. But I think she gets it more and more, especially now that she's going back to school to be a veterinarian. She's found *her* passion and I've never seen her so happy. Life is short and you have to do what you love to do every day.

It's easier to get away from the work than it is from the cancer. The cancer, it's always, "Where's the sunscreen, where's your wide-brimmed hat?" None of my friends are doing that. When I go play golf, usually I wear long pants. There's always a constant reminder. But on the flip side, I'm the only one that's happy when it's cloudy and rainy.

I think that, deep down, there are a couple of things that make me do what I do. One, I didn't have chemotherapy, so I sometimes feel like I didn't suffer as much as a lot of people, and here's my chance to give back. Two, chances are I'm going to have cancer again, and why not try to help as many people as possible now before that might happen? My chances are 75 percent for a recurrence of melanoma. Not to mention prostate cancer, colon cancer—I'm not planning on those anytime soon, but I would say that my goal is to live long enough to get prostate cancer!

I still have goals for myself. I really like writing and I have semi-launched a speaking career. I have a nagging goal of writing a book. I want to write something about cancer, but I want to focus on the activism side of it and really aim it at high school and college kids, proving that it doesn't matter how old you are, you can really have an impact and make a difference. If you have an idea, no matter what it is, and you think it's a void in your community or your area or your state or your country, go for it. Beyond cancer, it's more about making a difference.

One of the things I often struggle with is that I want to do everything NOW. I set a lot of year goals or six-month goals, but I don't set a lot of five-year, ten-year goals. Because too many things change, and I just want to concentrate on today. Sometimes I think it's hard for me to look that far in advance because I don't know what's gonna be going on. But I'm learning, especially at work. But me, personally, it's like, tomorrow? Where are we going? What are we doing for lunch?

I can't really remember what I was like before cancer because the last five years seem like twenty years. I've been through so much, it's like a whole new life. I was an athlete. I loved young people; I loved teaching. And I still do today. But I totally changed. Now it's different:

I just cannot stand to waste time. I can't stand when people are late if it's important, because there's just too much to do.

Three years after my diagnosis, I ran a hundred-mile marathon in the Himalayan Mountains with World TEAM Sports. I had never run more than eight miles at one time. I didn't know what I was trying to prove. I feared failure, and my thoughts ran through loneliness, death, fear, and uncertainty. But when I asked myself whether I would be able to complete the race, the answer was, "of course." I had been alone and nearly beaten before. As I hit the finish line after five days of running, I was overwhelmed with clarity. I felt incredibly alive.

Lance always says, "I wouldn't change it for the world." I always say that I wouldn't change it for the world, as long as I don't have to do it again.

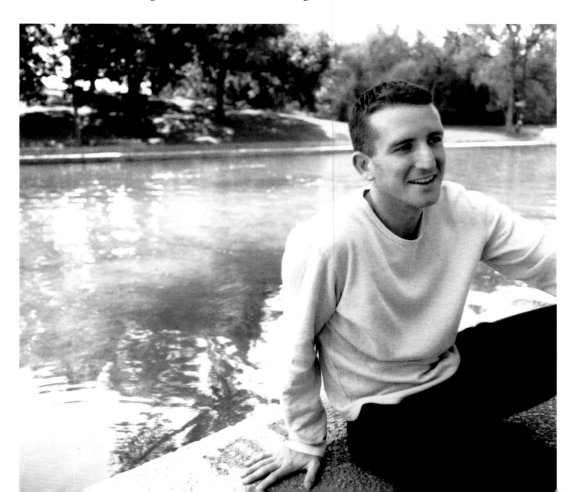

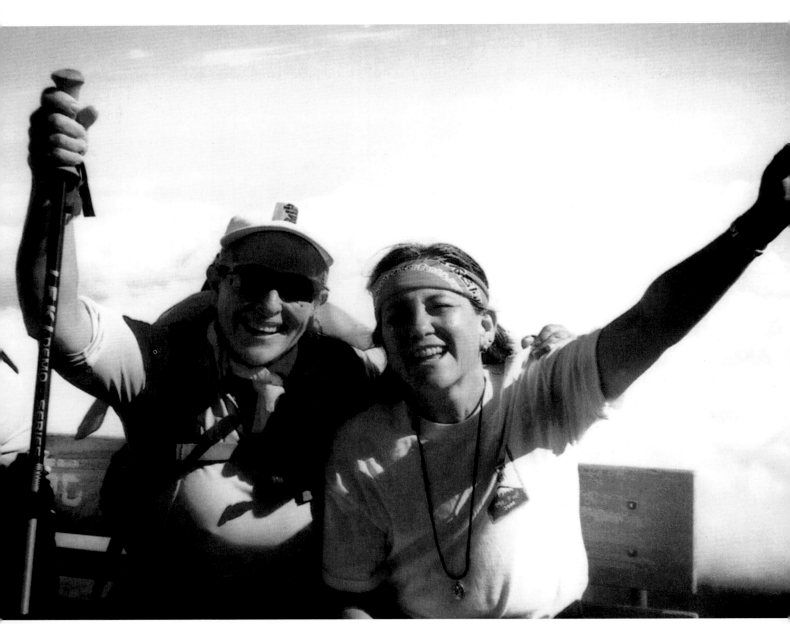

ANDREA MARTIN (RIGHT) *Photo courtesy of the Martin family.*

Andrea Martin

THIRTEEN-YEAR SURVIVOR
BREAST CANCER

■

*A*BOUT A YEAR before my diagnosis, my breast had started hurting. I had been told that breast cancer didn't hurt. To think that all the while I thought I was okay, cancer was growing in my breast.

I vowed to myself that I didn't care if it was benign, I was going to have it out. I never thought it was cancer. In retrospect, I was in a very strange depression shortly before and I had no real reason to be. I'd just married the dream man of my life. My daughter was doing fabulously. I was excited about my new career, which I was just formulating—service in women's issues. I'd been an attorney and just knew I wanted to do something to advance women's issues. I was just oddly depressed.

Of course I was. I was sitting there with stage 3B cancer. It was an extraordinarily, profoundly life-changing year. During that year, I was sure I was going to die. I had been told that my chances of surviving this were very low, and what they were doing was the most extreme treatment they could give me. My instincts also led me to reach out to all sorts of complementary therapies.

After my first treatment, I proceeded to throw up every minute for the next sixteen hours. I wanted to die. Afterward, I went to a holistic desert retreat. I was given homeopathic remedies for nausea, immune boosting, visualization help. Also, I got myself into a support group that was all women. All of us had been diagnosed within six months of one another, but I had the benefit of traveling down the road they had all been on.

I showed up at my second infusion and asked the doctor, before I allowed him to give it to me, what he was possibly thinking after that first one. Why didn't he give me Benadryl or Ativan? He said he wanted to see how I'd react and then he'd know what to do. You just want that person to have a bit of Adriamycin, cold, to see how they'd like it themselves.

Staring my daughter in her face was the hardest part. She knew her mom was sick. I wondered how I could convey to her, in a short period of time, all that I would want to say to her. I wrote in a journal to her. We brought her into the process as much as we thought she could understand and handle.

My support group that year lost seven of our fifteen members. That is not a statistical reality, but it was a reality for our group. I credit that, as much as anything, for the fact that I do the kind of work I do with women and cancer now. I had the privilege and the honor and the

I've always had a spiritual life, but cancer brought me levels beyond anything I'd experienced. I've always believed in the connection we have to our own wisdom. Cancer, and the work I've done since then, has opened up my thoughts in that regard even more. I now talk to thousands of women and tell them to trust their instincts.

responsibility in being present in the passing of these dear, new friends with whom I had very little in common except our journey with cancer. It had a very profound effect on me.

Maybe it was to bring me closer to what my real purpose in this life is. It was so intense and yet I couldn't turn my back on it. I think it is essential in healing to be able to talk and know that you are not alone; others are on the same path. The fears that wake you up in the middle of the night are fears shared by others.

I operated that year 100 percent on instinct. I've always had a spiritual life, but cancer brought me levels beyond anything I'd experienced. I've always believed in the connection we have to our own wisdom. Cancer, and the work I've done since then, has opened up my thoughts in that regard even more. I now talk to thousands of women and tell them to trust their instincts.

Women need to stand on their own wisdom when there is such confusion among the experts. We'd like to think the medical community knows everything when, in fact, they don't even come close. You have to be in touch with your instincts—in terms of breast cancer, it's probably the most protective element of your existence. I'd always trusted my instincts but never so much as after I had cancer.

A year after I was out of treatment, I was drawn into politics. I was named the northern California Deputy Finance Director for Dianne Feinstein's senate campaign. Two weeks later, I was brushing my teeth and feeling what was left of my breast, as I did all the time, and felt a tiny little pebble that I know wasn't there the day before. I waited two weeks and it did not go away.

Richard and I found that, a year and a half after finishing treatments, I had cancer in my remaining breast. I wanted the breast off. I grow cancer in my breast and I didn't want any more biopsies. Besides, I'd be symmetrical again!

We left the office and I was nothing but excited. It could have been a lot worse. It was a new primary, not a recurrence. I had a mastectomy and went back to work in two weeks. It was very different from the first time around.

But this is when the anger started. There are various stages of dealing with the threat to your own mortality and anger is one of the big ones. I really shifted from personal fear to being pissed off. Nobody was really talking about breast cancer or doing anything about it. Here I was, with no history of cancer in my family, feeling ambushed. I had been doing every-thing they told me to do and here I've had it twice.

There I was, in the middle of a campaign, having to approach life aggressively, and I gathered around me some of the smartest women I knew and started the Breast Cancer Fund. I finished out the campaign and began to grow the fund full-time. The Breast Cancer Fund was and is intended to push the edge on the issue; to constantly question the status quo, to provide seed funding for research and education and patient support and advocacy programs that are not getting funded anywhere else.

I think in the big picture, no one ever taught any of us to work together. I view breast cancer as a vehicle to actually help us learn how to step into our power as women, and how to learn to work together. The first few years of this movement have been getting into it, reacting to our urges to do something about this disease and, finally, finding our voice and picking out what we're going to do.

I'm really excited about the fact that I'm alive and I celebrate that daily. I am beating the odds at the moment. I would never say I have beaten the odds. My health is very important and foremost in a lot of the decisions I make. One of the things the fund stands for is ultimately increasing the odds for avoiding breast cancer and increasing the odds for longer survival.

The fund stands for wellness, for prevention, for more attention, for equal funding for prevention, and for study of environmental connections to the growing rates of cancer, as well as cure and treatment.

Personally, I am in the midst of major transformation in my life. I was never an outdoors person. But because of the fund I've become a bit of one. I have begun hiking and going down rivers, sleeping outside, putting up tents. I was part of the climb at Mount Aconcagua, Argentina; it was absolutely startling to me that I could do what I did and do it with a smile on my face. That was the first time I slept in a tent! In a very real way, I've taken on physical challenges. The activities of the fund come from my choosing some of the things I'd always wanted to do in my own life.

When a climber and survivor named Laura Evans asked the fund to sponsor her climb of Mt. Kilimanjaro for breast cancer, it dramatically catapulted us into this kind of activity, which I am extremely thankful for.

Physical activity—climbing—is a way to use the courage you uncovered fighting something scary, by doing something of your choice. It's already an incredible metaphor for going through the cancer journey itself, which is best done with the support of friends, taken one step at a time. If you look at the top of that mountain from the bottom, you can't imagine how you're going to ever get there. Well, how are we going to stop breast cancer? How are we going to clean up the environment? We're going to do it one step at a time.

Another unexpected, though welcome, path that I'm taking for my healing, is exploring my sensual path. When I was diagnosed, I was forty-two years old and newly married. Here I was, after my first chemo, thrown into chemical menopause when we were actually trying to have a child. After my first treatment I never had another period.

I was going through all the changes very suddenly and intensely. I got to a point where Richard wouldn't let me retreat or fade away sexually. Gently, he did the best he could to keep me in touch. As time went on, we settled into a part of our lives where I had absolutely no libido. It was as if it were totally stripped from me. It was sudden and horrible. Here I had this husband I lay next to every night and had nothing in me for him. If I had never had sex again, I would have been okay, or so I thought.

Well, knowing what I know now, that would have been suicide to part of my life force. I tried everything: chemicals, testosterone ground up as pills and cream, lubricants, other stuff, but it just wasn't happening. Finally, I attended a program that was a major step on my path to recovering my libido.

This disease is extremely tragic and we are losing women randomly. Women are being hit in the most vulnerable parts of our body. We want this to stop, as adaptable and courageous as we are. My biggest fear is that we will become too accepting of this disease. It's a wake-up to all of us. Because women are finding their power around breast cancer, we've got to use it as a wedge to change the way we walk on this earth.

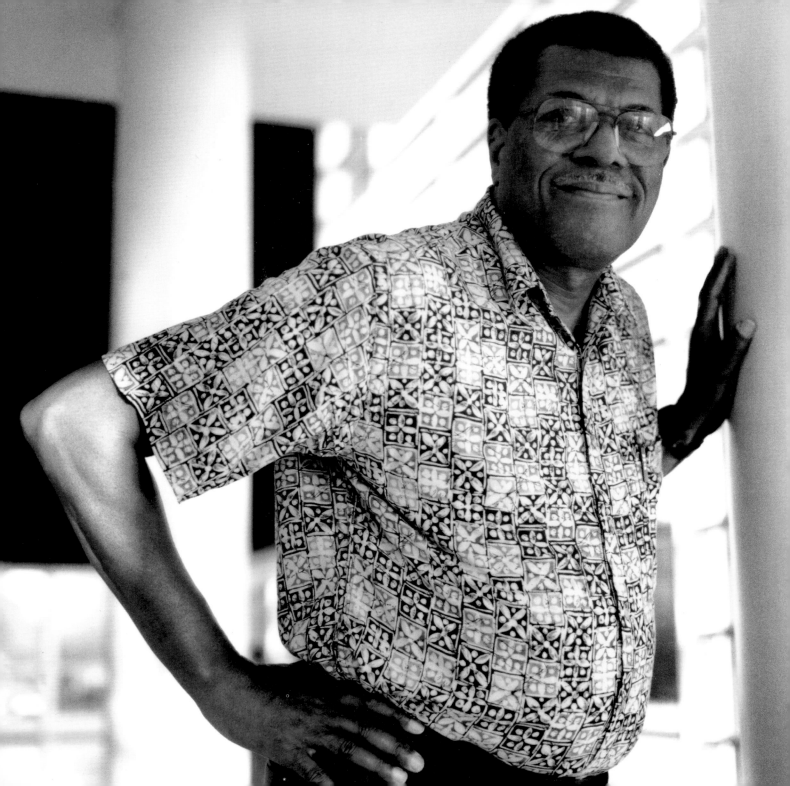

Ed Savage

SEVEN-YEAR SURVIVOR
PROSTATE CANCER

◼

*T*HE BIG "C"? I'm not afraid to face that guy now.

I had a lot of fear when I first found out. It was about seven years ago. The doctor gave me a rectal exam and he thought my prostate was excellent, but it turns out that my PSA was ten—normal is four or five. A few weeks later, it was twelve. I was blown away to know that I had the "C-word." The doctor told me, "You have cancer on the right and left side of your prostate. We'll remove the prostate altogether, but I'll try and spare a few nerves so you can still have some sexual feelings. Not a big deal." And he was showing me all these pumps and things. They looked like torture devices.

So then I started talking to people who had had treatment for prostate cancer. One of them was wearing a diaper for incontinence. The more people I talked to, I started saying to myself, "I don't know—I'm going to think twice about this surgery. There's got to be another way." So I called the doctor. He said, "Well, your surgery is tomorrow." And I said, "If I'm not there, start without me."

I'm a fighter, and I can't just sit around. I looked into all kinds of things. I started to look at natural healing and I found a naturopath doctor near my home. She had a machine that read the electrical impulses in my body, starting at my head and working down. She told me all about my family history, and I hadn't told her anything. She gave my wife a free exam and said, "You have scar tissue from a hysterectomy." We were blown away.

She mixed up herbs to match what was wrong with me and I tried them. Over the next eight or nine months, my PSA went down and down and down. She had also given me diet advice: go easy on red meat; eat fruits, grains, and vegetables—especially green ones—and drink things like carrot juice. We bought a juice machine and I was juicing, which does a lot of good. I had been a steak and potatoes man, so this was a drastic change. My wife helped me go through it and she joined me. As a result, her weight balanced out and if you saw her you wouldn't think she's sixty-four. I feel healthier and haven't had one minute's problem since then.

I bumped into my surgeon one day and he looked at me and said, "I'm disgusted." I asked why, and he said, "Because you look so disgustingly healthy." He said, "I don't know what you're doing, but keep doing it. Just don't tell me about it."

I run a group for people with cancer at my church. When we meet, we talk about our current status and treatments we're taking; people recommend treatments to each other. We're leaning a lot toward naturopathy because the side effects of some of the medications people are taking are horrific, so they're looking for other things.

At this point, if my cancer were to recur tomorrow and I couldn't get it under control, I think I could make my peace with God and be comfortable. I've had seven years—seven wonderful years, in fact. I think of it maybe a couple of times a month; it's always in the back of my mind. My wife says she thanks God for every moment I've had without having treatment problems and side effects.

I look at the medical community with a jaundiced eye now. I see the treatments that people are getting around me and I watch the mistakes that are being made. This business of the accountants running the medical systems at HMOs—doctors don't like it, but they have to work within the system. They rush patients; they don't send you for second opinions or follow-ups with specialists, just to save a buck. The cleanliness is not there now, either. A lot of people are getting staph infections in the hospital. Doctors are overworked and they're short-tempered. Our medical system needs to get back to where it used to be, when people were kind and gentle. I talk about this wherever I can and to whomever will listen.

My wife is my steadying hand to make me stick to what I'm supposed to do. Sometimes I slip, like when I see a big fat hamburger with cheese dripping down the sides. I'm not celibate; I gotta have one once in a while. My youngest child is okay with what I'm doing, but my older daughter, on the other hand, is relentless. Just recently she was after me about my health and how she didn't want to lose me. I told her I could step in front of a car. I tell her, "Enjoy me while you have me, hon."

This disease has increased my faith. I was raised in a religious family, but now my faith is deeper than it's ever been. There's definitely a connection between not only faith but frame of mind. It's so important to be positive and that's what I preach to people who are sick. I know you're afraid and everything, but be positive. I tell people to try to get out in the sunshine. You always feel better when the sun shines on you.

I bumped into my surgeon one day and he looked at me and said, "I'm disgusted." I asked why, and he said, "Because you look so disgustingly healthy." He said, "I don't know what you're doing, but keep doing it. Just don't tell me about it."

My son got married last weekend. I think I danced too much. My sister likes to dance, too, and I told her, "You're going to have to realize that we're in our sixties. We can't cut a rug like we used to!" I'm still able to run. I think about those things and count my blessings. Every day I wake up I'm extremely grateful. Even if it's foggy and ugly, it's still a beautiful day to me 'cause I'm here.

Next month I'll have been married forty-one years, and my marriage is just as sweet as it could ever be. My wife and I hold hands. We kiss three or four times a day, and we hold each other at

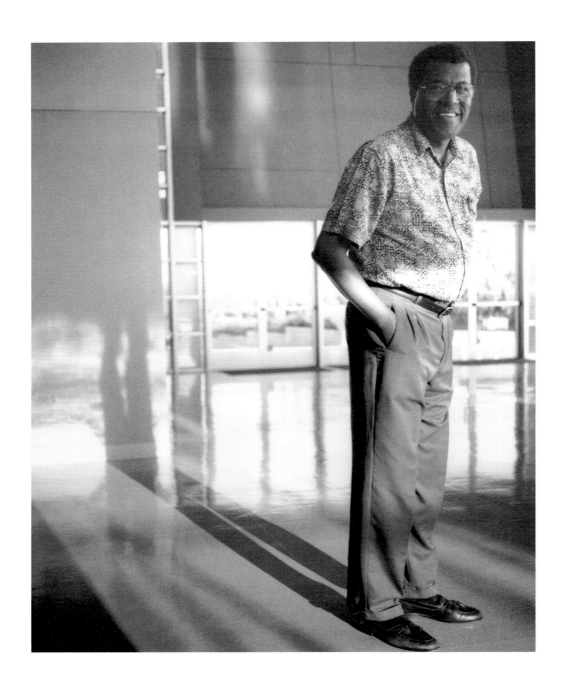

night; it's really nice. We've always been close, but more so now and we're both appreciative of the time we have together. We're not just husband and wife, we're friends, and that's important. I try to give advice to young people to be appreciative of their girlfriends and spouses, and to treat them right. Hopefully some of it will rub off because life is too short to be the way I see some people are.

I wouldn't want to be the person I was before. I'm more patient. I'm not selfish anymore or self-centered. I'm open to everybody now; it's not just about me. I don't care about keeping up with the Joneses. I used to want a nice car and to have the latest of everything, but I don't worry about it anymore. Life is just too precious to even worry about material things. I worry about my health and other people's health now.

I know now that people have to take charge of their own health. Even if you go with conventional medicine, you've got to look at who's treating you and what they're doing, and if you're not satisfied with how things are going, get out. I know some doctors are very good. My support group has an oncologist that comes and speaks; he's a very good doctor and he respects my opinion. He never belittles me for what I think. But some people have bad experiences and they just stay there.

In the next few years, I want to try to help as many people as I can get well without them getting sliced and diced. You know, if people want to have surgery, that's fine. If that's what they're comfortable with and they think they can tolerate it, fine. I still think that, if you're not in real serious straits and you have time, you should try to cleanse yourself and leave yourself together. Get alternative help from somebody who knows what they're doing. I consult with my doctor and I feel strong and healthy, but who's to say? It's in the hands of God.

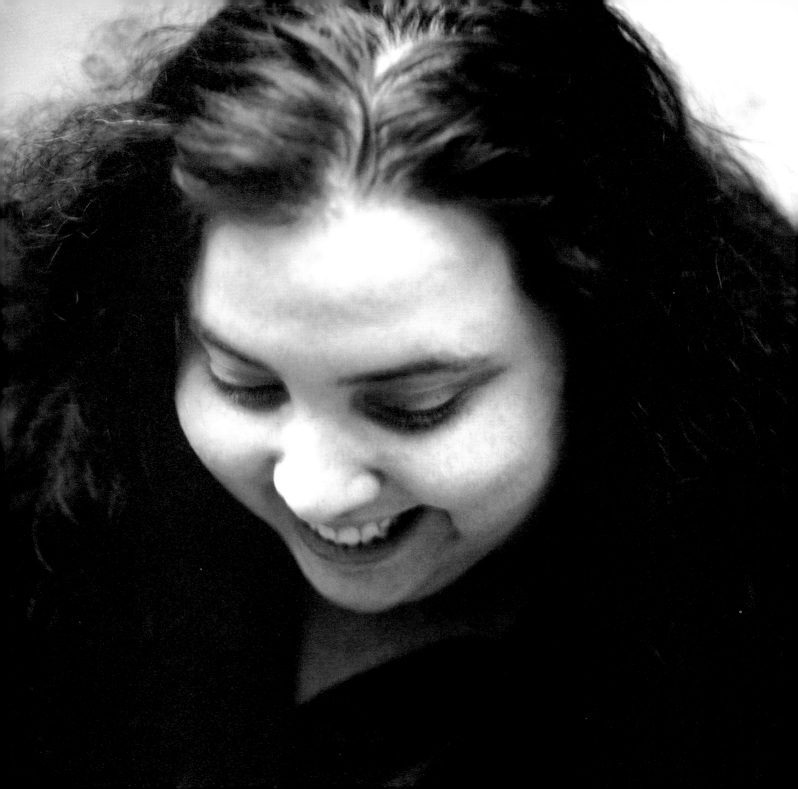

Juliette Forstenzer

TWO-YEAR SURVIVOR
UTERINE CANCER

*I*HAD BEEN in therapy twice a week for maybe six years, struggling with bulimia and self-mutilation and all sorts of obsessive-compulsive stuff. When I was diagnosed, all the areas that I thought I'd recovered from, like my sense that my body is my enemy, just came roaring back.

My periods had been irregular for many years. Finally, I had a D & C and they found an unusual amount of polyps in my uterus. The doctor called me at work and said, "You have stage I uterine cancer. You're going to be okay, but we need to take some immediate action." It felt like I was in a bad movie. After that, my sister and some friends came over to my apartment and we got drunk. Every time the phone rang, my sister would pick it up and say, "Julie can't answer. She has cancer."

I had a partial hysterectomy, so I have my ovaries, but I lost my uterus and cervix. I didn't need additional treatment beyond surgery. My first reaction was to blame myself and turn my anger inward. My brain couldn't even comprehend the permanent consequences from the hysterectomy. It got stuck on having this weird guilt because I hadn't been through chemo and radiation. I didn't feel like I belonged with healthy people or with sick people. I had also lost my connection to the whole cultural web of being a woman: the whole birth control thing, dealing with your period, all the things that you learn to negotiate in your twenties. I would go into the grocery store and get incredibly upset if I had to walk down the tampon aisle.

The first year I was in a state of complete shock, trying to get by day to day. I was drinking and smoking pot. All I wanted to do was check out. After my one-year anniversary CAT scan, I decided that I wanted to try and take control over my life. I got sober and started getting crazy about eating healthy, like all the orange and green foods. I got really into the treadmill.

I was setting up my second-year anniversary CAT scan when, one day, there was all this blood in my stool. I had a colonoscopy done, and they found four polyps. I felt like I was having a flashback. It was like the entire two years came crashing down on me. I was totally convinced that I was sick again. I was like, fuck it. There's no need for me to be sober. I need to have a drink and be left the fuck alone; to isolate myself and freak out about this.

It hit me that I would never *not* have a cancer history; that the doctors would always be hypervigilant with symptoms that might mean nothing in others. I remembered my blissful ignorance of my own mortality in a very potent way, and was overwhelmed with sadness because I'd never have it back. Then I had a moment of clarity. It happened in a flash—I just got brave or something. I said, "You know what? If I'm sick, I'll deal with it. I was sick before, and I'm alive to tell about it." I decided that sitting in my apartment getting wasted was in no way a good choice for me, no matter what. I got sober and started counting days again in AA.

The colonoscopy results were completely innocuous; everything was fine. But a week after that, my sister's periods started getting irregular. She had been like clockwork her whole life but, because of her family history—meaning me, since there was no other history of cancer in my family—they decided to do a D & C to take some cells from her uterus for a biopsy. She was diagnosed with endometrial hyperplasia, which is a tendency for the uterus to build up excess lining. Most likely, it ran in our family, and the reason I had gotten cancer was because the lining had built up for so long. The doctor told her outright, "The fact that your sister developed uterine cancer is going to prevent you from developing it." It was just this really powerful thing for me. It allowed me to give meaning to the fact that I had had cancer, and changed my sense that I was just a freaky person with a freaky body.

I got so many gifts from getting sick, especially in terms of reconciling with my body and how to care for myself. I remember when I was fourteen or fifteen, I really believed that I could get a body transplant—that I could get my head put on someone else's body. I carried that into my twenties because I had so many body issues. The cancer was like a sledgehammer to my skull, saying "This is your body!" Cancer has brought me back to my body, but in a brutal way.

The entire process was an accelerated maturity. I have reestablished my relationship with my parents in a way that is much healthier. I'm able to recognize how much I've changed my perspective, my priorities, and the way I cope with terror and grief. I'm much less harsh on myself and on other people. If people can't rise to the occasion when I need them, or if I feel like I'm not strong enough to show up for someone, emotionally, then I'm able to realize that that just happens sometimes. I'm much less judgmental.

My sister thought that when I was diagnosed I would kill myself or OD because I was such a depressed person. Instead, my reaction was fierce, like, "I will do whatever I have to do to be okay" because, suddenly, I didn't have the luxury of choice.

The way that I relate to people is different. I frequently end up talking about really personal things with people I've just met. I think it's because I've become so blunt and honest about my own stuff that people feel comfortable to be honest and open back. Before, I came from a place of shame about who I was. Having had cancer is so essentially a part of who I am now, that I'm not going to hide it. That openness about cancer seeped into other areas, which has been a big change.

The best coping mechanism I learned was to take actions that feel good to me and that make me feel less powerless. No one is in charge of what the end result is going to be. I'm not in charge of whether or not I get cancer again. But I've been shown so many times the things

I *can't* control, that I became aware of the things that I *can* control, like making good food choices or arranging my apartment the way I want it.

Right after I got sick, my family started an adoption fund for me. At first I didn't want anything to do with it, but now I know that I'm going to adopt kids. I have three friends who are pregnant now and it's hard because I'm jealous. I feel like, "Oh, I'm going to have to come up with $20,000 and prove that I'm an okay person before I can have a kid, and you just had to go get laid." How is that fair?

I have a master's degree in gender studies and feminist theory with a focus on medical history but, even with my level of consciousness, I felt disempowered when I was ill. When you're ill, you're vulnerable, yet you have to do your strongest advocacy for yourself. I'd like to help people through that. I've done some work with the Leukemia Society in terms of health insurance legislation and the rights of cancer survivors. I'm looking into starting a nonprofit and opening post-treatment centers in other cities.

My sister thought that when I was diagnosed I would kill myself or OD because I was such a depressed person. Instead, my reaction was fierce, like, "I will do whatever I have to do to be okay" because, suddenly, I didn't have the luxury of choice.

Is everything the way I want it to be? No. Do I feel good all of the time? No. Do I have plenty of issues that I need to work on within myself? Absolutely. But I feel like I have energy to do it in a way that I didn't before, and I feel like I have an attitude that allows for possibilities. Those are gifts from having cancer. How could this terrible thing that makes me grieve, that terrorizes me, also have provided this whole way of being? That's kinda fucked up! That's where the maturity comes from because, as you mature, you learn to deal with paradox.

I was talking with my sister one day, and she asked what I would say in a VH-I "Behind the Music" about my life. I told her that I wasn't going to have a "Behind the Music," that I was going to have a biography on the Biography Channel. And they would talk about "the life-changing experience of when she had cancer, during that short period of time when she foolishly worked in corporate advertising." So I'm hoping that I live a long and fascinating life and that I end up on the Biography Channel.

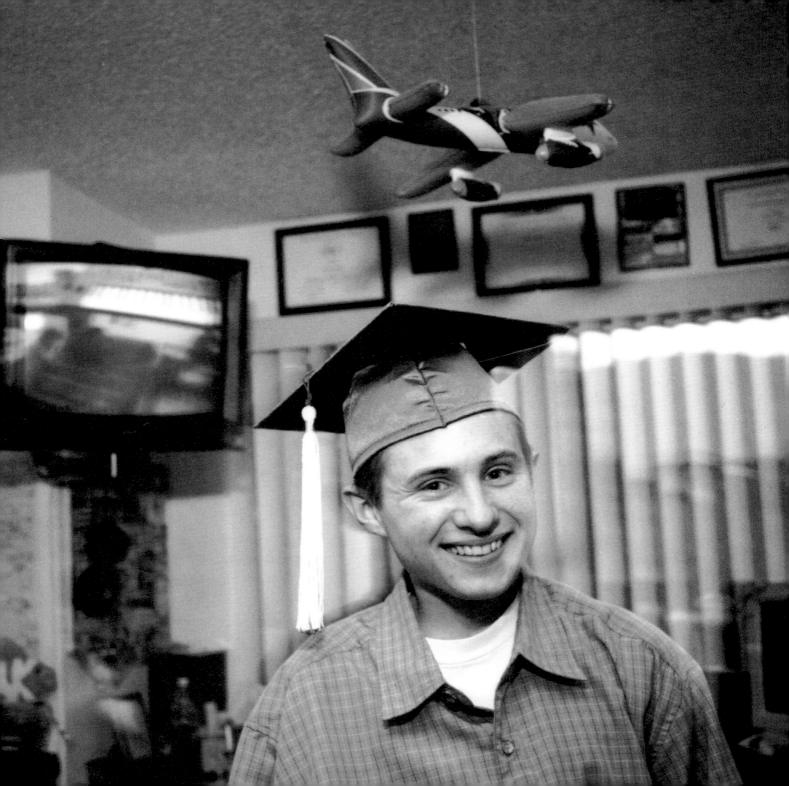

Drew Hiben

PARENTS: *Andy and Lesa Hiben*

TEN-YEAR SURVIVOR

ANAPLASTIC
ASTROCYTOMA

I HAD BEEN feeling kind of weird, and one of my hands was bigger than the other—that's how we first noticed it, when I was eight. There was a tumor in the spinal cord that was blocking the blood flow to the right side of my body. It's called anaplastic astrocytoma and is actually a brain tumor, but it showed up in my spine.

When I had the surgery, I thought my head was going to fall off. They had to take out the bones in my neck and rewire them. So for the longest time I was afraid to let go of my head because I thought it would roll off. After that I had chemo, which was just an all-night puke parade. I remember the bone marrow transplant tasted like garlic when they injected me.

LESA: *The doctors were saying they weren't getting the results they wanted, and there was no history to go with, because there weren't a lot of kids with tumors in their spinal cords. They had no information to go on. When Andy and I decided to put Drew in a bone marrow transplant, we literally shook hands and made a pact. We actually said, "If we are standing over his grave, together, we're gonna hold hands. We're not going to say, 'What if?'" And that was it.*

I don't go around telling people my story, but when people see my scars, they'll ask. I guess it's kind of impressive. I don't walk around saying, "I SURVIVED CANCER." You kind of save it for the right time. And then, it's kind of like all inspirational, I guess. When people ask, it really makes me think about why I'm here now, but it's not something I dwell on.

It was fun being in the hospital. I made all these friends, and I felt safe there. When I had to go home it was the worst day. My parents had changed my room because they had to clean it to get rid of any germs. So I was in this new room and then there was an earthquake, and I felt like my house was going to fall down on top of me. I was crying because I wanted to go back to the hospital.

My best friend in the hospital was Daukari, who also had a bone marrow transplant. We went home on the same day. Daukari and I always talked about destroying the hospital and building an amusement park over it. But then he relapsed, and we didn't really talk about it any more. Even though we didn't live together anymore in the hospital, we were supposed to get better and carry on with our lives. And then, all of a sudden, that wasn't the case. It just wasn't fair. But I don't think about him much anymore. I kind of moved on with my life.

LESA: *I noticed the difference in his hands, therefore, "It's Mom's fault that I had cancer." And I will take that with me to my grave! With his neck surgery, it was, "Mom keeps up with the MRIs and Mom says, 'Oh, doctor, do you notice such and such?"" And then he has to have surgery and wear a halo. So he's very selective about what he'll tell me. He knows that my radar is immediately on.*

ANDY: *He'll tell me a lot more, especially when it turns to guy stuff. When he was young, especially being on chemo, your body's open to the public. Nothing is sacred. As he got older, he's like, "Mom, leave the room. Dad, I've got a rash on my butt," or something like that. I guess it happens to all teenage boys; they get to that point where it's kind of a guy thing. And that hit really quick for Drew.*

Because they had radiated the bones in my neck when I was first treated, it was growing funky, so they had to straighten it out when I was sixteen. The doctor said we were going to have to fuse my neck, and I would have a big halo with bolts in my head. That was the worst. I was supposed to wear this halo for three months, but I told the doctor, "You have three weeks, and then it's coming off." And when I went for my checkup after three weeks, everything was looking good, so all I had to do is wear one of those things that looked like I got in a car accident. I heal myself really fast. I drank a lot of milk.

When I'm determined to do something, I'll get it done. I've always been a success story, though. I was the doctor's guinea pig in the hospital for my bone marrow transplant, because it was so experimental at the time. It gave me the mentality like, I'm a winner. I can do anything.

I don't go around telling people my story, but when people see my scars, they'll ask. I guess it's kind of impressive. I don't walk around saying, "I SURVIVED CANCER." You kind of save it for the right time. And then, it's kind of like all inspirational, I guess. When people ask, it really makes me think about why I'm here now, but it's not something I dwell on.

ANDY: *Drew doesn't want to be made into a hero for surviving cancer. When he sat down and wrote an essay for this cancer thing where he got some scholarship money for college, he didn't have to put a lot of work into it, he just wrote his life story. I think he's feeling unworthy of the honor and recognition he's received for it. We keep trying to tell him that this is a combination of everything he's strived for in his academic career. But he is my hero. This kid is awesome. The way he goes after things and accomplishes his tasks is something that I really try to live up to.*

I realize now how lucky I really am to have survived something where the odds were so against me. Worse odds than in Vegas. They said the first surgery was like taking chewing gum out of my hair, because the tumor was lodged in my spinal cord. I can move my legs now. I can walk. There was a pretty good chance that I wasn't gonna ever do those things again. Or that I wouldn't even wake up.

I'm more proactive instead of just sitting back and letting things happen. I have a reason to go out and do something with myself. I was dormant for a period of time and now I'm so active in school—I'm thirteenth in my class, out of seven hundred kids. Recently I've become more of a risk taker. I might as well try new things.

I'm going to college this fall about an hour away. I'm living on campus in a dorm. It should be interesting, because I have this chronic fear of pooping, but that's another story! I think cancer has made me more of a private person. Since that time, I've always liked to be alone. I don't like to talk much about myself, because I feel like I'm more in control of me. And that I'm more powerful. I never was one to share my emotions, especially in the hospital. I always kept everything to myself. It was a pride thing.

> ANDY: *Drew was always doing something like the Boy Scouts or playing outside, but after this happened, he became kind of a loner, in a sense, even though he does go out and has a great group of friends. I think a lot of it was because he had so much attention brought at him with the nurses and the doctors and someone always asking "How are you feeling?" or "How are you doing?" He likes to spend time alone now.*

I think my experience made me want to go into a service occupation. Not like a priest or anything—I want to be a teacher. A lot of people that go through treatment are like, "I want to be a doctor." That won't work for me. I don't like blood at all. I didn't even take biology— I took physics instead. Blech. I could go into a high-paying profession or something, but I feel like I'm going into something that I love and that I believe in.

The experience definitely made me closer to my parents. We're very close, 'cause it's just the three of us. Mom was the caregiver, I was the strong one, and my dad was in the middle, holding us in balance. Mom's the one that always tried to make me careful. She's still like that. I'm eighteen and she's still treating me like I have a lump in my spinal cord. But she just cares a lot, and it doesn't cause any problems.

> ANDY AND LESA: *We have an only child—an only child with a history of cancer, and we've been through so much together, it's almost twice as hard to let go. I've noticed that experiences like what we went through either tear a family apart or bring them closer together. We pulled on each other's strength and created a bond between the three*

of us. We learned to take the little things and celebrate them. On his second birthday—the anniversary of the transplant—we celebrate the strength and the fortitude and love of the three of us. But this year, we kind of forgot about Drew's second birthday. I think it's a transition. There are so many anniversary dates that you can associate with negativity that we made a conscious decision to stop doing that. I think the flip side is just to celebrate the joy of each day.

He makes us want to be better people. The way we relate to life, the way we treat others. Drew would go out and move a bug before you could squash it, just because it needs to have an opportunity to complete its life cycle.

I'm more apt to see the different ways and the different meanings that something can have. It's like those gardenias outside the door, I always stop and look at those. They smell so good! But that's not the only thing. It's made me realize that there are phases in life and right now it's warm outside and, when I stop and smell the flowers, it's kind of nice to be alive.

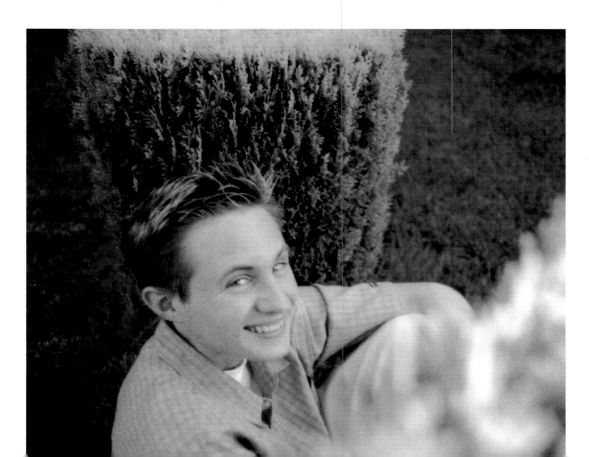

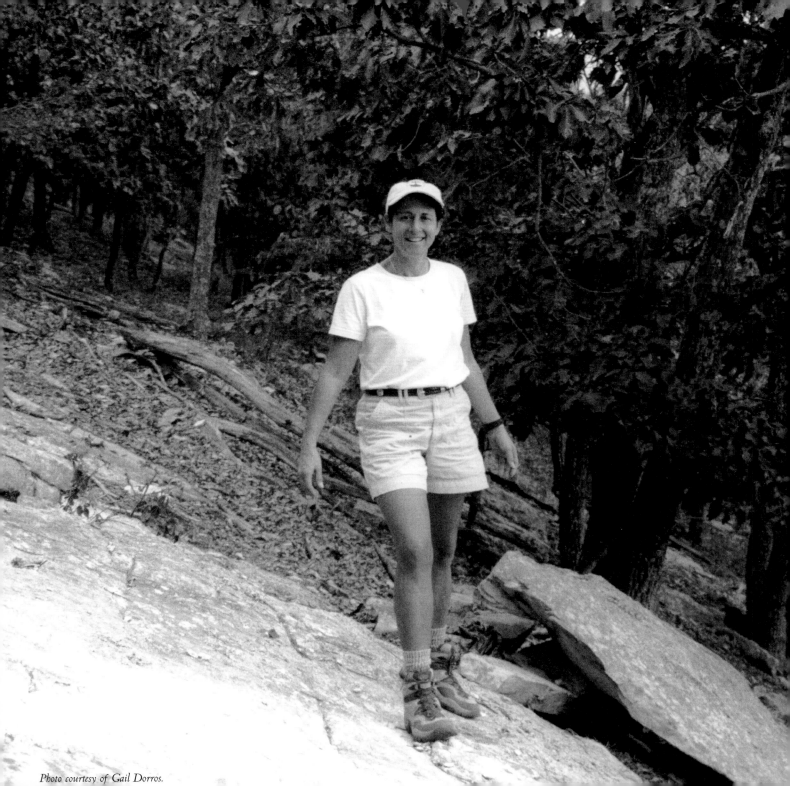

Photo courtesy of Gail Dorros.

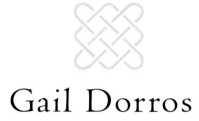

Gail Dorros

SIX-YEAR SURVIVOR
BREAST CANCER

I WASN'T AWARE how seemingly common it is for women who have just given birth to have breast cancer. My gynecologist did not examine my breasts, so I didn't pay attention at that time. I knew my breasts were going through many changes being pregnant, but I just didn't worry about it.

I was originally diagnosed in August of '95, when I had a mastectomy and reconstruction. I wanted reconstruction right away, so I wouldn't have to deal with the idea of not having a breast.

At the beginning of 1996, I felt a lump in the same area where they had found the cancer and done the reconstruction. The doctors thought it was a fatty deposit, but I insisted they take it out. It was a recurrence.

I found a new team of doctors, including a *breast* surgeon, which was something I should have done the first time. I had the entire reconstruction and more lymph nodes taken out, plus a hysterectomy. They put me on tamoxifen and gave me radiation. I knew I wanted to have more children but, at that point, I just wanted to survive. I stopped working and I joined a support group.

For about a year, I wasn't comfortable with being naked or making love. I've lost that over time. Arthur doesn't even bat an eyelash. He tells me he loves me for who I am, not my breast. That has been huge for me. It's hard to tell my daughter. She sees me naked and she wants to touch my prosthesis. I tell her that most women have two breasts. I also tell her that it is private. At the same time, I don't really mind if people know. Then we can joke about it and not have it as a source of strangeness between us.

When I was first diagnosed, it never *really* got to me, deep down. I didn't cry. I just did what I needed to do. I went to my job four days a week. I didn't want this cancer to take over my life. I even got a promotion while on chemotherapy.

When the cancer came back, I felt like I was punched in the stomach. I needed to do something else. Up to that point, I had the "white cloak" syndrome—whatever the doctor tells me, I'm going to believe and do. I had done a ton of research myself and always had many different opinions, but all within the traditional realms. This time, I started incorporating alternative reading into my life and found a doctor who knew a lot about nutrition. I switched my diet completely to follow his plan.

Ultimately, I felt total responsibility to make the choices—and the right choices. I had wonderful support, but I was on my own. It was incredibly frustrating to talk to the people who you believed knew what to do, and they didn't. One doctor actually flipped a coin. Stuff I'd taken as gospel I just didn't anymore.

Most recently, I had a chest wall occurrence. I was ready to have them tell me more chemotherapy and maybe a stem-cell transplant, but they told me I should just watch and wait. They put me on a new hormone treatment. I asked myself, "What can I do?" That's when I started high-gearing into alternatives.

I took time off from work to get my head in gear, which was hard to do. I had a lot of guilt around, "Do I really deserve to be on disability? Do I deserve the time off?" But I just knew I needed to do it. I didn't want to keep going through the motions of my life. I got on the Internet and found many trials going on that I would be a good candidate for. To hear that there were more choices on the horizon was really encouraging. I didn't take any action at the time, but I wasn't closing a door; I was just waiting, investigating both Western and Eastern treatment options.

I began to work with a Korean healer who is skilled with herbs and teas, acupuncture, and meditation. Through meditation, I've learned to zero in on my feelings and talk about them. I ask myself, "How do I feel, right at this moment?" That's wonderfully calming. I've also started yoga, which is putting me more in touch with my body sensations.

The spots on my chest went away. I believe it was due to the teas and all the work I was doing. The Korean healer has taught me to not fight the cancer. Someone has to win, and you get tired. When cancer emerges, it wants a home in your body. We go after it to kill it, and it fights back. Changing the environment so it doesn't want to be there anymore is what I'm after. Not trying to fight the cancer, but to build myself up.

My daughter is my biggest salvation in this, but she's also my biggest source of pain. I desperately wanted to have children. She is my main reason for wanting to live. I am so thankful for each year we have together. I try and make sure that I'm in every picture with her that's taken, so she will at least have that if something happens to me.

I've been given the gift of knowing that life is short and a gift from God. If someone gave you a gift of one hundred dollars, you would say "Thank you," not "Why didn't you give me a thousand?" Short or long, I'm thankful for my life.

I'm not by any means thankful that I had cancer. But I've discovered that life is a journey and that's exciting. I've been given the gift of knowing that life is short and a gift from God. If someone gave you a gift of one hundred dollars, you would say "Thank you," not "Why didn't you give me a thousand?" Short or long, I'm thankful for my life. Cancer has opened up so much to me that I never would have done, and I find it fascinating. If it weren't for the fact that it could kill me, it would be quite interesting!

I've found some pledges that help me now: "I accept. I forgive. I'm totally reconciled to everything. I'm satisfied." The first time around I dealt with the physical, the second time with the mental, and the third time was to teach me something about my spirituality. Once I was able to realize what spirituality is, I was able to know that I am a spiritual person. I got in touch with a whole part of myself that I was unaware of before.

I discovered that I had defenses for suppressing feelings that were ingrained from childhood. Someone once asked me in college how I felt about things, and I didn't even know how to answer the question. Now, when I'm feeling something like sadness or anger, I consciously let it come out.

I'm speaking from my heart more. I'm also learning how to trust myself and not look to others for answers. I've learned to question everything, to be my own advocate, no matter what! People in the medical community make mistakes constantly. I wasn't aware of that before.

I'm doing all this nontraditional stuff, but there is a mainstream world out there and I've got a mainstream family. I'm trying to figure out how to transform so I can be healed but stay connected to what I love and am familiar with. It helps to be around people who feel the same

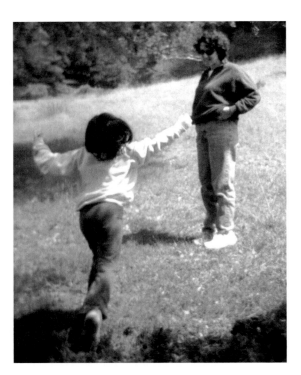

way, but much of my journey has been solo because it involves personal exploration. I try to share some of my experiences with my family. Sometimes they get it, sometimes they don't. I like when people ask me about cancer or my alternative practices. Then I can share and teach them something they may not have had the chance to try.

I always assumed that everyone with cancer would view the world the same as I do, so I was amazed that nearly half the people in my support group were on antidepressants. I'm in such a different place than most of them. Take charge. Be active. Don't complain. That's my philosophy. People ask me how I'm so strong; I think that, when it's handed to you, you make the best of what you've got. But it doesn't mean I'm not angry about my losses: not being able to have more children, loss of body parts, the carefree lifestyle.

I find that as much as I don't want to know what will happen, I know I will face it and go on. One of the things I've learned is not to spend energy on what I can't change, but on what I can. That is enormously comforting. I can only lead by example and this is the kind of example I'd like to be: do what I can every day and stay unattached to how things should or shouldn't be. Awareness is the first step toward a better life.

I'd like to survive the next ten years. I love birthdays and I love getting older. I'd like to see my daughter bat mitzvahed. It seems like a great reality that I will be around for more of her life. I'm at the tip of my spiritual journey now and I feel that is just beginning. I'd like to be able to get to the place where I can make a mark by helping other people—not necessarily with cancer, but with healthful living in general. I want to have fun. I had always wanted to know true love and to have a child. I've gotten those things.

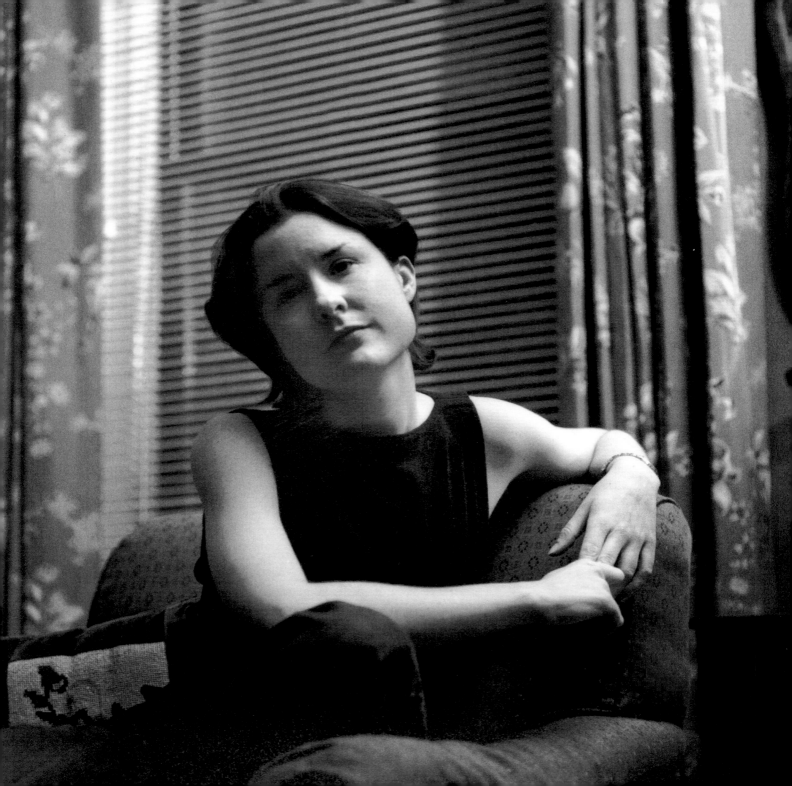

Megan Olden

TWO-YEAR SURVIVOR
HODGKIN'S DISEASE

I GUESS I had been sick for a while, but I didn't pay attention to the details: fevers, strange skin things, weight loss. And I had this lump on my neck, about jawbreaker size. I was at the doctor's for another reason and I asked him to just confirm that this thing on my neck was nothing. And he touched it and said, "Oh, my God. Hang tight." He came back in two seconds and announced, "We gotta remove this."

I went home and sobbed for a long time. I tried to imagine them saying that I had cancer and what that would be like. What I would do. I imagined that I would go for a drive and, dramatically, it would all become clear. After the biopsy, I found out that it was Hodgkin's disease.

At this time in my life, I was just about to take a huge leap and move to New York City to launch my national magazine career. I was working as an associate editor for a small medical trade publication in California, and I had finally summoned the gumption and the funds to leave. Instead, I had to go back to the job I had just quit and say, "I beg you. I don't really want to quit. I want to stay—and do chemotherapy." They said okay.

I like to make informed decisions so I went and got tons and tons of medical journal articles. I felt like my life was at stake and it was my responsibility to educate myself and figure out what to do. I didn't trust that somebody else was going to have the right answer. My boyfriend was a lot of help in making decisions because he was a medical resident at the time.

I felt freakishly out of control and really wanted to regain some of that. I wanted to have some kind of power in this situation. I quit therapy because I felt like I had to get through it on my own. I didn't really want to analyze or feel sorry for myself—I already felt like I was terribly overanalytical. I just had to put my head down and go through it. I got a lot of support when I finally told my friends and family that I had Hodgkin's.

I'd always had the experience that if you put yourself out there—if you really throw yourself out there with a lot of passionate energy—good things happen to you. After the diagnosis, these illusions were shattered.

My boyfriend and I were trying to figure out how to navigate our relationship. I needed him so much, but I couldn't really be angry with him for not being there, because he was taking care of other sick people. He was my touchstone as to whether my medical team was being honest with me. He called every day and tried to see me twice a week, which was huge and really hard for him to do with his schedule, but it wasn't much, considering how frightened I was. He took a lot of the terror out of it for me, but sometimes I think he felt like he knew what I was experiencing better than I did. When I wanted to go out mountain biking or do crazy, wild, active things on the good days early on—because that already felt so precious to me—he would say, "You could hit your head and have a subdural hematoma." So sometimes I just wished I was dating a carpenter!

I booked a weekend at a B and B and spent extravagant amounts of money on spontaneous gestures of joy like that, especially in the beginning. I dragged my boyfriend off to Napa; hired a masseuse for both of us, things that we couldn't really afford. But suddenly saving money seemed a little ridiculous. I had always been future-oriented, which suddenly felt very flawed. I felt like maybe I needed to learn to maximize my enjoyment now.

When I was in treatment, I didn't want to move to New York anymore. I just wanted to go to a beach house and lie around for a while. And everyone said, "You have to get back on the horse and you can't give up your dreams and this can't beat you." So I came. But I kind of regretted coming. When I got here, I still couldn't walk up a flight of stairs without resting, and I didn't feel like fighting the big fight.

So here I am in New York. I have a sense of mortality now. I want to slow down and really be good to myself, and yet that feels at odds with getting ahead, especially here. I want to have a garden and I want to pet my dog—which I don't have, but I want to get a dog, and pet it! How do you come to terms with living in the moment, yet planning for the future?

The one-year remission thing was a huge release for me. After I was declared in remission, I felt like I had to be aware at all times, so I would never be surprised again. I've lost my sense of invincibility. I'm aware that terrible things can happen at random, like bus accidents and cancer. Somehow the surprise had been the hardest part. I checked my lymph nodes daily. I went to the doctor and they asked me if I did monthly breast exams; I said, "I do them every day!" I used to prepare myself for them to say it had returned. Now, two years out of treatment, I've watched the fear diminish greatly. I haven't forgotten about cancer, but it's sort of way in the back of my mind.

When I was sick, I'd drive down Highway 280 toward Stanford and the light would be a certain way, and I'd start bawling in the car. I'd get down there and my boyfriend would think I'd lost my mind, because I'd just be like, "It was so beautiful!" I think things touch me deeper now. People don't get that. They don't get it at all.

When I was sick, I really felt I needed my friends. I tried to tell them what my experience was like, but I felt that they just had no idea what I was really going through. Some people didn't talk to me at all, some people acted like I had the flu, some people acted like I'd already died. For most of my friends, it was completely foreign. None of them had the sense of vulnerability I have.

I didn't write at all when I was sick, I just kept a journal. I started taking notes not long out of treatment, but even that made me nauseated. I did write down some sensory details and the texture of things, so that I would have them later when I had some distance. I tried to write an essay about having a "good" cancer, which was just very weird. It was strange to be told over and over how fortunate I was to have Hodgkin's; sort of this strange win-the-lottery sense.

I know I am really lucky. I think when something like this happens, it gives you something back. Right now I'm training for the Team In Training marathon, to raise money for lymphoma and leukemia. It's the kind of thing I could motivate myself to run twenty-six miles for—one of the *only* things. Almost every time I run, I feel how exciting it is to be strong. It feels great to be out there, running, watching the seasons.

I experience the preciousness of things more than I might have before. I still have the same personality traits, but I question more. Being hard on myself makes less sense. Today, I am not willing to put myself through a lot of things, emotionally, that I used to think would spur me to greater achievement. I'm still pretty driven, but it's shifted. When a new job offer came up recently, it was exactly the kind of job I would have gone for, yet it would have involved moving again, a $20,000 pay cut, working really late. Before, I would have done all that just for the job— no questions asked. But I declined the job offer. I feel good about that.

I booked a weekend at a B and B and spent extravagant amounts of money on spontaneous gestures of joy like that, especially in the beginning. I dragged my boyfriend off to Napa; hired a masseuse for both of us, things that we couldn't really afford. But suddenly saving money seemed a little ridiculous. I had always been future-oriented, which suddenly felt very flawed.

When I was in treatment, I slept on a futon. I vowed to myself that I would never, ever sleep on a futon again. And that I would never, ever have an apartment that didn't feel like a haven to me. I have a lovely, full-sized bed in my lovely brownstone in Brooklyn that overlooks a park. It is a good change. Before, home was something that I used as a launching pad for other things. My life was about quantity. Now, it's more about quality. I'm really trying to make things count. I'm cultivating fewer friendships, but am there more for the friends I have. I write less, but I write better. I want to do things that would have felt like failure before, like settle down and carve out a life for myself.

Cancer feels like an important event in my life. This thing was not a little bump in the road, it was a detour. I don't want cancer to always be this huge traumatic, Top Two event of my life. Right now it's more of a central event than I wish it was, but I know that is temporary. I want to take the lessons from this and keep them with me, because otherwise, what was it for? Not that it had to happen but, otherwise, there's no point to the hard parts. I mean, I can write a couple of good short stories with really telling details, but that's not enough to justify it. I know in some way it's helped me evolve faster than I might have, and I'm trying to learn how I integrate those things into my almost-thirty-year-old life.

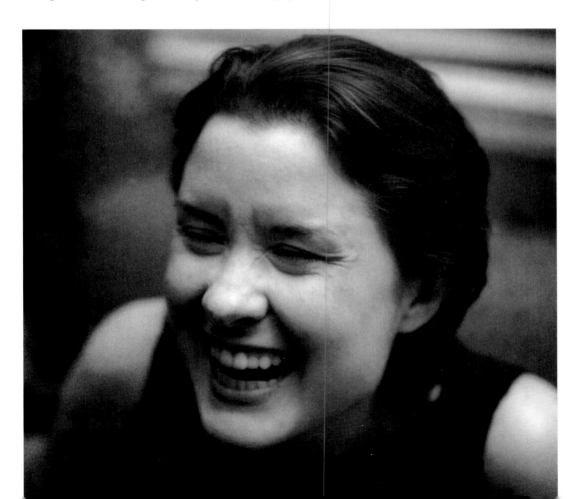

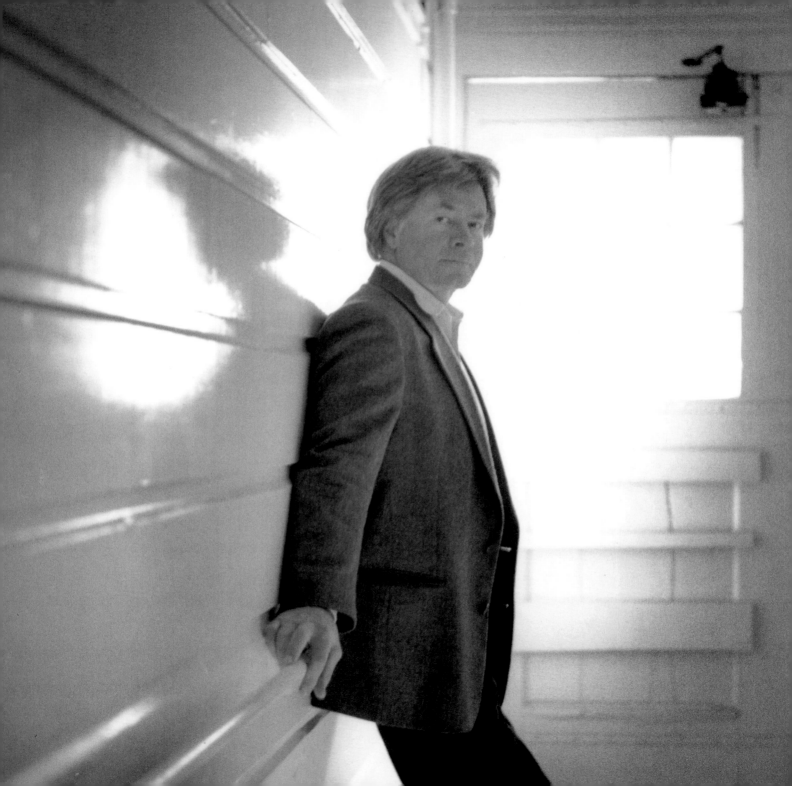

Mark Dowie

THIRTEEN-YEAR SURVIVOR
ACOUSTIC NEUROMA

*I*N 1985 I had a tumor in my head that was cancerous. That was shocking news. I found out by listening to my watch that I could hear the ticking in one ear and not the other. It seemed that something between the inner ear and the brain was a problem. This wasn't one of those hideous tumors which spreads through the brain like wildfire; in fact, the doctors told me I could wait almost a year before the surgery had to be done. I didn't know how to tell my wife,

Wendy. I was very concerned about it, but when I got home, she knew. I walked in the door and she said, "You've got a tumor, don't you?"

I began to do my research over the next few months. I found a great library that had all the lay materials and obscure stuff and I became as sophisticated as I could about the anatomy, the terms, the surgical techniques, the chemistry, and the history of the epidemiology. I didn't understand the intricacies, of course, but I was able to converse with the doctors. Once I'd done the research, I started looking for the right person to do the surgery.

I found the best people were right here in San Francisco. I still had to ask them: "How many have you done? What's your success rate? How many acoustic nerves have you lost? How many facial nerves have you lost?" A very high-powered microscope and laser scalpel were used for my surgery. They removed the tumor one cell at a time with a tiny laser knife. I had always been a bit of a Luddite, but I can't ignore the fact that I was saved by extremely advanced technology.

The idea of time is the gift I've taken with me from this whole experience. The thought of getting and having more of it. You have to look at time in a mathematical way—that it is something you have that is yours and yours alone. It has a finite quantity.

I knew, when I was being wheeled down the hall, having said goodbye to my wife, that this might be the last time. My kids were grown and living their own lives. I was only forty-seven—I was too young for this. But in some respect, I got myself ready to die.

Wendy was fantastic during my illness. She stayed in constant touch with my entire family. She put long messages on her machine, updated every day, with news of how I was. She was by my side all the time she was needed.

After the experience, I started rebuilding my life pretty quickly. I was very, very tired, but once I was at home I felt as if I could begin to heal. It took a long time before I had more than two to three hours a day of working energy. The steroids I was on created a crazy euphoria. And nobody warned me about it! They didn't think to tell my wife, either.

Wendy tells me almost once a week that I'm a better person since all this happened. I'm more understanding. I know that compassion and love and kindness are essential to life. Because of my experiences I have become a lay counselor to brain tumor patients. I try to tell them things that I would like to have known: How to look for information, where to get good literature, what to look for in a doctor and so on. I think I offer a sense of hope.

It feels so good to be back, to hear the doctors say, "It's going to be okay, you'll live a long life." As time goes on, the recurrence curve drops off; I've now passed my tenth year. And of course, I knew deep down, from the very beginning, that this would not be the thing that killed me.

The idea of time is the gift I've taken with me from this whole experience. The thought of getting and having more of it. You have to look at time in a mathematical way—that it is something you have that is yours and yours alone. It has a finite quantity. I've always appreciated trees, nature, life eternal, life force, and the miracle of life. But I always thought the gift of life was something that I received forty-seven years ago. You know, you can waste almost everything and recover it. Money. Friends. But the one thing you can never recover is time. My attitude toward time now is reflected in a refusal to do anything that doesn't have meaning to me. I get a lot of offers to work, but most of them I'll turn down. Sometimes I look at the bills piling up on the side of my desk and think I had better take the assignment. But I don't.

Subsequent to all of this, I inadvertently became a Buddhist. I practice in some form every day. Part of the practice is to learn to separate the things you have control over from the things you have no control over every minute of the day. One can learn to accept the inevitability of death, the beauty and reality of death.

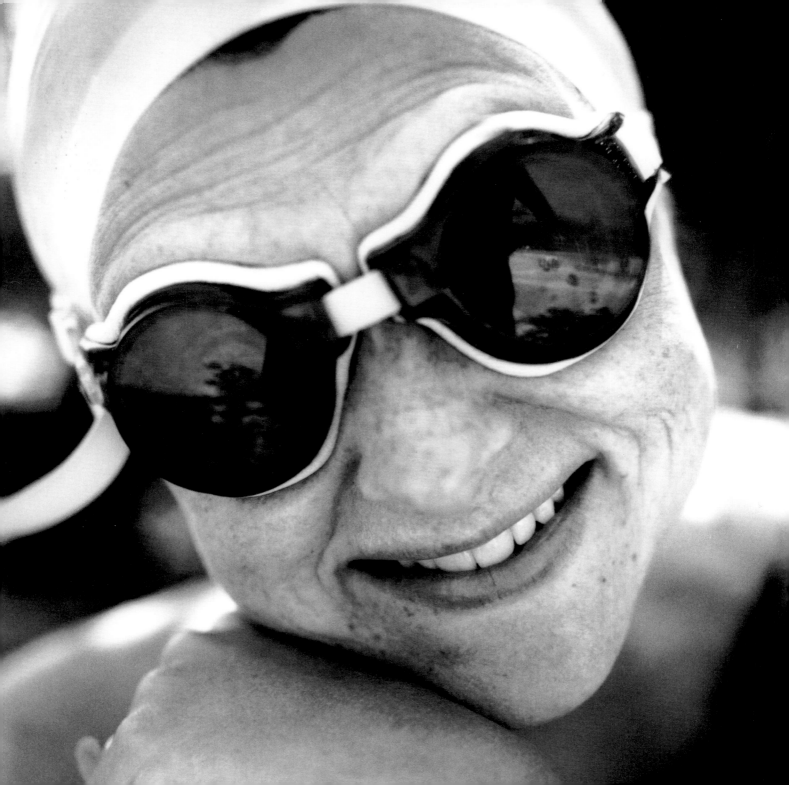

Susan Taylor

TWENTY-THREE-YEAR
SURVIVOR

HODGKIN'S DISEASE

I GREW UP in Maine. I was a competitive synchronized

swimmer and was accepted to swim out in California. I moved

to the Bay Area as a college freshman. Middle of November,

I started having chest pains in the pool. I had a chest X-ray,

and they found a tumor in the heart area. My doctor sent me

to have a biopsy, where I was then told I had Hodgkin's.

My mom came right out when she heard. My family was getting advice like, "Bring her home and let her die here, in Maine." It was really horrible. But when she came out to Stanford, she saw a lot of hope there.

I had total-body radiation therapy, from the chin down, for three or four months. That's the way they did it then. That was '78. I managed to stay in school. I went back to swimming. I jumped in the pool and did two strokes and thought, "My God, what have they done to me?"

In March of '81, I had my follow-up at Stanford. I went to the hospital feeling fine. All of my other follow-ups had been great. I said to my boyfriend Martin, who is now my husband, "I'll just go by myself. It won't take long." That was the wrong thing to do. There was team of doctors standing around looking really sad, which scared the life out of me. I had a recurrence. Dr. Kaplan said, looking down at the floor, "Treatment is going to be really different this time." He meant chemo. I remember thinking that I was not going to die, but I was petrified of chemo because I'd seen what it did to people.

I was scared and shocked. My first semester in college, I was diagnosed for the first time. My first semester at my transfer school, I was diagnosed again. I thought to myself, "I am never going to another college in my life!"

I was crying and I called Martin. He was great and supportive. I met him at a Halloween dance in college. Love at first sight. I knew he was the guy for me. We started dating in the middle of November and I got the news of my cancer in early December. Martin spoke to a nurse who told him that she really believed that I was going to get better. In those days there wasn't a whole lot of hope. We'd never heard of anybody surviving cancer, so what she said had a real effect. Martin wanted to stay with me, even though our relationship was so new. He decided he wanted to help me get better. If it wasn't for that nurse, he probably would have left me. I don't know if I would have made it without him.

When I was diagnosed, I was incredibly strong and fit. I felt great. I think that was a big plus for getting well. But things were way, way different the second time around. My mom flew out again. We were all pretty shook up. The doctors told me to drop out of school, so I did. My biopsy was really deep in the chest. It was a horrible thing to go through. After the operation, Martin basically took care of me in the hospital.

At the time, I was living by myself in Palo Alto. My mom, who is like Miss Victorian, came into the hospital one day and said, "I've thought about it, and I think Martin is the best person to take care of you. I'm going to have him call his parents to ask if he can move in with you." I nearly fell over. Wow! That's when I knew the cancer was serious.

I spent my days lying in bed. One day turned into the next. I stared at my Maine clock for hours. I didn't even realize that I was in a really deep state of meditation. I started hearing this voice, which later told me that it wanted to be called my Creator. I thought it was God speaking to me.

This voice told me that there was a reason why I was where I was at, and that someday I would do something special. I knew that if I just got through treatments, things would be fine. And that is true today. That helped to keep me going through that very dark time. I was afraid to tell anybody about it. Even when I got better the voice continued, and it does today. The voice is like my guardian angel or a spirit guide.

I believe I was sick for a specific reason. It was to be able to give to other people the lessons I've learned. It was also for my soul's development. But I had to go through a hard time to learn. I didn't cave in, although I came awfully close.

I was depressed for years afterward. I was depressed about losing my swimming career. That was big for me. Occasionally, I'd get angry at my limitations, but I just wanted to live. One minute I was really strong, and the next, very weak. I didn't know if I should or even could plan five years ahead. I didn't know how. I thought I could be diagnosed again at any time and I didn't know what they could possibly do for me if I were. I was so worried. I was certain that there was no way I could do chemo again.

Over time, the fear of recurrence went away. I don't live with it anymore. In '83 I started going to the survivor group for Hodgkin's that was created at Stanford. Everybody was scared of recurrence. We talked a lot

I have a four-page handout that I give to every new doctor, because it took too long for me to tell my history. They love it. No matter what doctor appointments I have, I take all my medications with me to show them. The handout has all my major history and doctors listed with names, phone numbers, and addresses. I update it regularly. I didn't do this for them, I did it for me.

about side effects. I found it fascinating and helpful to listen to other people. They were saying the same things I'd been afraid of.

I finished college in '85 and then I began working on the survivor's newsletter. I also began editing a magazine about survivors as an offshoot from the group. We realized we had something to say. Ultimately, I became the managing editor. It was fantastic. I could have an editorial board meeting and feel relaxed. I wouldn't even associate my cancer with those meetings. I can separate the two very easily now. It just happened naturally.

I live differently from my friends and people who haven't had a life-threatening illness. When I had chemo, I was in bed for nine months. I remember thinking, "When I feel better, I'm going to be excited to get out of bed every day." It's been years and I still feel that way!

If I plan to do something, it means a lot to me. I make a point of telling myself to really look forward to it, to really enjoy being there. And to think about the event afterward. To reflect on it. I make things a big deal. I remember the times I couldn't do special things, so I don't take anything for granted.

I don't understand the people who have survived cancer and sit home all day in the chair watching TV. They feel they've been though something and they don't ever have to put themselves in a risky situation again. I've become more goal-oriented since my illness. I'm ready to challenge myself. Cancer comes in and out of your life. You just go on.

My husband and I really hate the residuals that cancer has brought on today. I have two to three doctor appointments a month and it's really stressful. These are directly due to my being sick. It's been happening more and more as I get older. If I get sick—and I do a lot because my immune system is weak—I go straight to bed. It can be weeks that I stay there. It takes all my energy to take care of myself. It's hard on both of us.

I have a four-page handout that I give to every new doctor, because it took too long for me to tell my history. They love it. No matter what doctor appointments I have, I take all my medications with me to show them. The handout has all my major history and doctors listed with names, phone numbers, and addresses. I update it regularly. I didn't do this for them, I did it for me.

I think of myself as a survivor. Meaning that I went through something that many people have died from. I know that I'm not ready to die because there are an awful lot of things for me to do. One day I was around the house and I turned on Oprah. She said, "Today, we're talking about why you are on this planet." All these memories came back about when I was sick. Now, I feel I was created to put down my experiences on paper.

I'd really like to see my book published. And I'm excited about swimming again. I can't wait to be forty! I remember thinking at eighteen, "If I can only make it to twenty, that would be great." And here I'm going to be forty. If you told me in the hospital that I would make it to forty, I might have lived very differently. I think about that a lot. I've overdone it this decade because I'm scared time is going to run out. I keep telling my Creator not to take me yet; there are things I want to do.

If I make it to fifty, it will be very exciting, and wonderful things will happen. I see that as a good time. It's my feeling. I hope I'm in good health. Ten years is pretty fast.

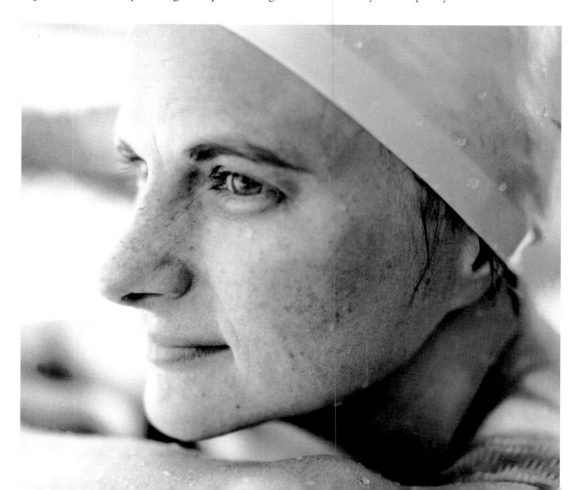

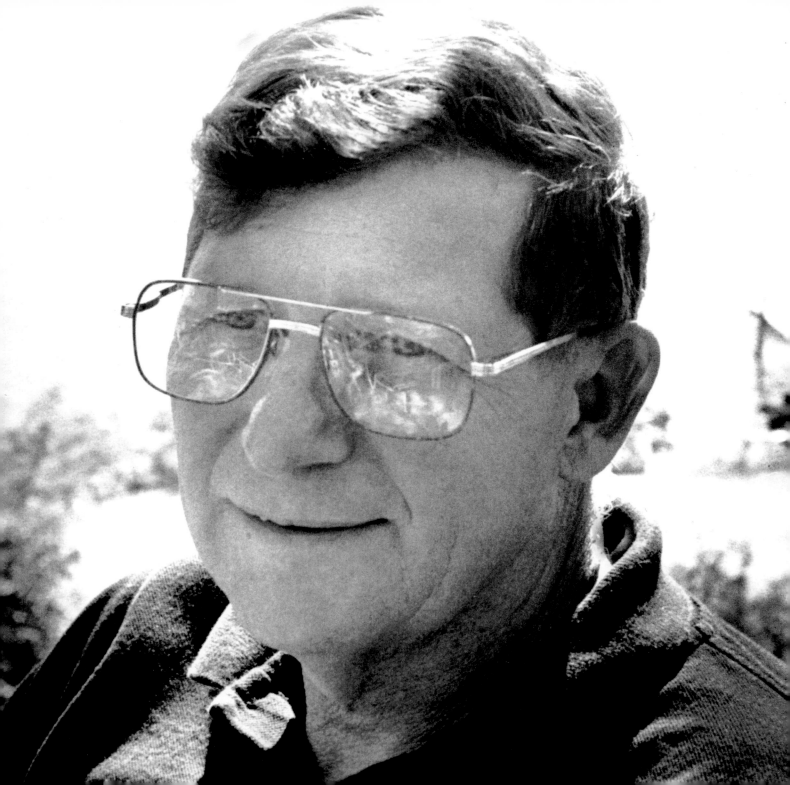

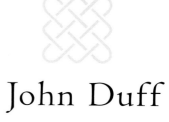

John Duff

SIX-YEAR SURVIVOR
MULTIPLE MYELOMA

*I*KNOW THAT I got my cancer from Agent Orange in Vietnam. It's a defoliant, developed in the forties for farmers. It's a major pesticide and it's very effective. We were in the middle of the jungle and we used it to kill all the bush around us so no one could sneak up. In April of '68 and '69, my troops sprayed it every day. We didn't have any protection—just sprayed it everywhere. We were covered head to toe in it every day.

In the early seventies I started to have bone pain; sometimes in the hands, sometimes in the elbows. It was diagnosed as arthritis but, as the years went on, I had difficulty getting up in the morning and walking. By '95, it became apparent that I had something other than arthritis. We had gone back and forth with the Army hospital. I said I had a problem, they said it was all in my head. We finally did an MRI and within ten minutes they found I had a three-inch tumor in my spinal column. I had multiple myeloma throughout my body, eating my bones away. Over the years, I'd had broken ribs for no reason at all and no one ever picked it up as a problem. That's a classic sign.

In '95 I had spinal-cord surgery to remove the tumor and five vertebrae. I had a couple months of radiation. They talked of a bone marrow transplant then, but wanted to wait until I became "sicker." Later, they determined I should have the transplant when I was feeling good, not sick, so I started a regimen of chemo for a few months.

I had to go to Nashville because the VA does bone marrow transplants in only three locations. After much conversation—and being approved by the Transplant People of the World, in Washington—we went down there from Boston. I'd been in contact with transplant support groups online, so I had talked to people who knew the places where there were empty beds.

I got to Nashville in August of '96, where they took out bone marrow and stem cells, and I had total body radiation. They also gave me more chemo and I had my marrow given back in early September. By the end of October I wasn't doing well. I was living off of transfusions and I had never left the unit. I wanted them to give me back my stem cells but it was too early, according to the protocol. I knew I'd be dead if I waited. I signed a release. Within days my counts started to come back up. It brought the cancer back, because the stem cells were taken before I'd had my final chemo and radiation. But I've survived.

I've learned a lot about medicine. I can't say my care was always good, but I've always been a special case. They say myelomas are significant with Vietnam vets. There are more than forty cancers tied to Agent Orange, but most people don't know that Agent Orange causes cancer. All you have to do is look in the paper and see vets dying, usually around age forty or fifty. You can see the code words: "died after a long illness," or "been retired for ten years."

When I retired from the Army I was a colonel. I had a retirement physical, and when the doctor told me that no one has died from the chemicals we sprayed, I told him, "Bullshit." He said the Army didn't use it, but I had gallons of it at any time on my ammo dump. It makes me angry to see people dying and kids who have lost their parents. The Army betrayed the troops, but they just try to wear you down until you stop making noise.

That's one of my missions in life, to keep talking. I talk to everyone about Agent Orange; I go on the Internet and help anyone I can. There are about 2.5 million veterans who were exposed to it, and only 250,000 vets have had Agent Orange screening. The Army is not doing a good job of letting people know about the potential effects, and I think it's done on purpose. I get government compensation each month, 100 percent disability. They have probably spent over $500,000 on me to date, but they will only help vets when it's absolutely forced on them.

Right now I'm taking experimental interferon three times a week at low levels, and I take meds to prevent thrush and shingles. I do the interferon at home, myself. My wife, Margie, measures it and I do the injection. I put out my pills every morning like a ritual. My mother was ninety when she was doing the same thing; here I am at fifty-seven and I have become my mother! I have bloodwork once a month, but that's it.

Today, it looks like there is nothing wrong with me. I have no bone pain. Overall, I know things are good. I know my limitations. I gave up work because I don't have the energy. I take a lot of naps on my desk at home. We just got back from a thirty-two-state, 10,000-mile trip. I had my fortieth class reunion a few weeks ago, and I was voted "Least Changed!" The chemo got rid of my gray hair.

Once, in the beginning, a doctor said to me, "They are going to come in and tell you that you are going to die. You just tell them you want a bone marrow transplant." I had no idea what that was. They all came in and told me I was going to die within seven months, that I had incurable multiple myeloma. I kept repeating, "I want a bone marrow transplant, I want a bone marrow transplant." I didn't even know what it was! Had I not told them that, they wouldn't have given me the option. It's all about money with the Army.

There are more than forty cancers tied to Agent Orange, but most people don't know that Agent Orange causes cancer. All you have to do is look in the paper and see vets dying, usually around age forty or fifty. You can see the code words: "died after a long illness," or "been retired for ten years."

I've learned that the transplant was the right decision. It's not for everyone; it's a personal, high-risk decision. You have to have a positive attitude and faith. A lot of people just give up. My wife challenged me the most. She was my cheerleader in Nashville. She watched over me all the time. She made sure the doctors paid attention to what they were doing. She helped me get out of bed and shower and ride the bike like I was supposed to. We've been together twenty-eight years and we knew what we were getting into. She never once thought I wasn't going to come home with her. I had wonderful family and the support of friends. There is no question that all the people around me made a difference.

Earlier in my life I thought the government wouldn't do anything bad to me. When I was in the Army I would have denied all of this, just like everyone else. But now that I'm out and something has happened to me, it's my mission to bring it out in the open. I am too young to die and I have too much to do. I'd rather die trying.

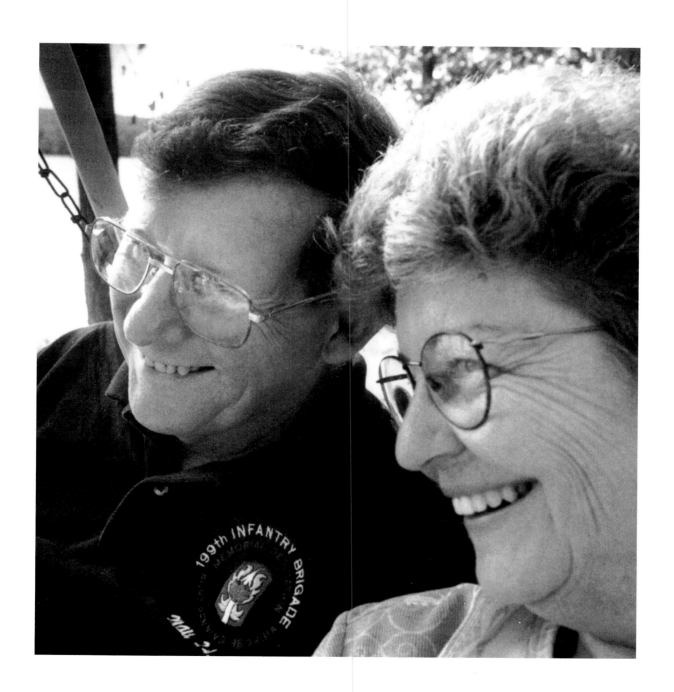

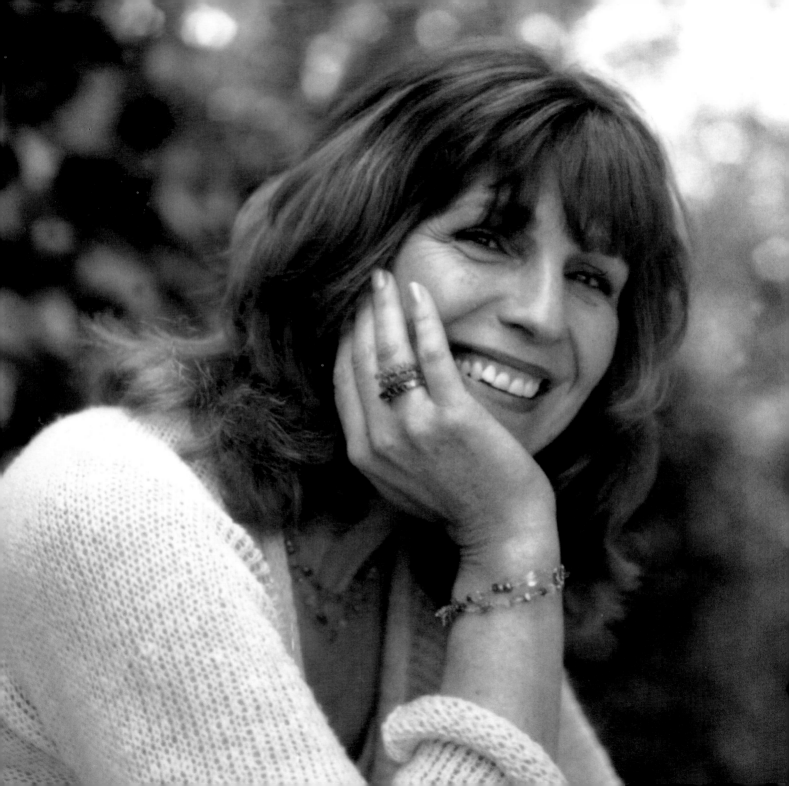

Julie Dresner

THIRTEEN-YEAR
SURVIVOR

HODGKIN'S DISEASE

■

I WORKED AS a stylist for the TV show *Night Court*. I was tired a lot, but I figured, I've got a little kid and I'm working. I'd always been really healthy. What sent me to the doctor was that I developed an odd kind of itching, like in my veins. I thought maybe I was allergic to something.

It took nearly two years to diagnose the Hodgkin's. After I started chemo, I continued to work, but I only told a few people I was close to about the cancer. I didn't want a lot of people to know. It was shame and embarrassment, the humiliation that something so horrible could happen to me. I was afraid of judgment from other people.

I was thirty-eight and my daughter was three. My therapy for myself was to just keep life as close to normal as I could to try and minimize the cancer. Chemo was just one more thing I needed to do in my busy, busy week. I never stopped for a minute to change my life in any way.

After a while, though, I began to realize how driven I was; how possessed and compulsive about having order and control. I started to recognize that I needed a way to cope, and I got involved with Chinese medicine. I started taking a class in visualization and meditation; started seeing a therapist. But I still never felt well. I felt weak. I got pregnant again but I couldn't have the baby. It was a tough time. Through it all, I continued to work.

A year and a half after I finished chemo, the Hodgkin's came back. I started treatment again, only this time I decided I wasn't going to work. I was going to really take the time to look after myself. My daughter was now five, and old enough that I had to talk with her about my illness. I told her that I was sick; that the medicine that was going to make me well was going to make me a little bit sick, and my hair was going to fall out. I didn't sugar-coat it and we didn't talk about it behind closed doors. We faced it honestly with her and I said, "I'm not going to keep talking about this to you, so if you have questions for me, you come and talk to me about it." We kind of left the ball in her court and she asked some questions, but not many.

One of my strongest memories from that time was a moment when Paul, my husband, was playing with our daughter. I could see into the kitchen and he had her up on the counter and they were giggling and laughing. Suddenly, I saw myself out of the picture. And I saw that they would be fine, whether I was there or not. I had a certain peace because I thought, I want to be here, but if I'm not, they'll be okay. And that peace has stayed with me ever since.

When I first started doing all this meditating and getting involved in Chinese medicine, I was very selective over who I told. At first I was embarrassed and ashamed, because some people would look at me strange, poke fun at me, call me woo-woo and New Age. But slowly I began to expose myself. I realized that the shame was causing more problems than the judgment would have.

Judgment has been a big issue for me for most of my life. I started to slowly realize that what anybody else thought about me had no bearing on my life, what my life would become, or what my outcome would be. I started letting go of the shame, letting go of the humilia-tion, the embarrassment of it, and I started telling more people that I had cancer. Now, I can't know somebody without them knowing that I had cancer, because it's who I am. If you're gonna be my friend, you have to know I am a cancer survivor. I'm very proud of it.

I decided not to go back to work in TV. I knew that era of my life was over. It was time to go on and do something else, even though I was getting calls to work and I was turning down huge amounts of money. I'd walk around the house going, "Oh, my God. I can't believe I'm doing this!" But I had sworn to myself that if I could be well, I wouldn't drive myself and worry about money.

When I was diagnosed for the third time, I had completely changed my life. It was almost eight years after the last time; close to ten years from the first occurrence. I had stopped working, I was committed to looking after myself and to living in a beautiful, calming environment. I had started my own jewelry business so I could work out of my house. If I was tired I would rest. If I was energetic I would work. I could work out, I could have time to meditate, time to eat right and sleep when I needed to. I could be a stay-at-home mom. I could take care of my family.

I always had my own little theories as to why I got sick, and I think a lot of it was that I was striving for things that were just not aligned with my soul. My body wasn't set up to push in the way I had pushed. I used adrenaline all my life. When I didn't have the energy, I went into my adrenaline reserves; I became almost an adrenaline junkie. As I slowly began to get it, things slowly began to shift.

The last go-round with the Hodgkin's was the most interesting. And as much as I learned through all of them, I think I really got the lesson with that one. It was really rare: not in the lymph system, not in a major organ, just sitting there like a pimple under the skin on my chest. My doctor presented my case to a committee of the top Hodgkin's doctors in the country and they all sat around scratching their heads.

For the first time I thought, you know what? If this is so rare, if all these experts don't know what to do, I'm gonna make the decision I think is best. I've done everything they've said in the past, I've done all the treatments and more, all the Chinese medicine, all the mental work, all the soul-searching, everything. I'm really gonna make my own decision on this. I decided I was comfortable doing low-dose radiation to the site. Since then, I have never felt better in my entire life.

It felt great to take the reins, although it was scary because it was my ass on the line. But I knew my body, I knew my emotions, I knew that I had no guarantees anyway. I feel like I'm buying time until Avon comes out with its Cancer Be Gone spray. I'm so much stronger than I was thirteen years ago. I have so much more energy because I've learned how *not* to use my reserves. I've learned how to be my real, authentic self. So I feel very satisfied with my choice, and I'm willing to live with whatever complications arise because of my decisions.

Before, I didn't have a lot of self-worth. I knew I was really good in a lot of ways: I was a nice person, talented and intelligent, but I always needed other people to remind me of that. And I think the switch is certain age wisdom, certain illness wisdom, certain spiritual wisdom from a lot of places.

My relationship with my husband has gone through so many metamorphoses that it's pretty astounding that we're still together. And I love him so much more now than I did at the beginning. When I was diagnosed, he took me to treatments, cleaned up the vomit, changed our daughter, loved her, never broke down, never wavered, never for a minute did he think that I was not going to make it. I was just astounded that somebody could really love me that deeply and support me so much.

Then our relationship went through a really difficult time and I had to make a decision about whether or not to stay in it. I remembered everything he did for me, and I thought, "How can I leave him at a difficult time in his life?" I decided that I was going to commit to this and do whatever it took. We've become different people but, through it all, we've become more committed to each other.

What I still strive for and ask for every day is, "Dear God, how may I better align with my soul?" I think that it's helped me to reach out to other people. At a very young age I felt a big responsibility to give back, so now I want to have the time and the health and the vitality and the wisdom to be able to do that on a topic that I know a lot about.

Now I really work under the assumption that I'm fine. I'm a huge planner. My plan is just to keep buying myself five more years. It's all in how you choose to look at it. My perception can make my reality. That applies to any aspect of life. Even just the reality of getting older. I turned fifty last summer, so that's been a real changing point for me. Look at me—I'm fifty and I've done all this stuff. I've had this amazing life and I've battled back from the cancer dragon three times. I'm healthy and I'm fit and I feel better than ever.

It felt great to take the reins, although it was scary because it was my ass on the line. But I knew my body, I knew my emotions, I knew that I had no guarantees anyway. I feel like I'm buying time until Avon comes out with its Cancer Be Gone spray.

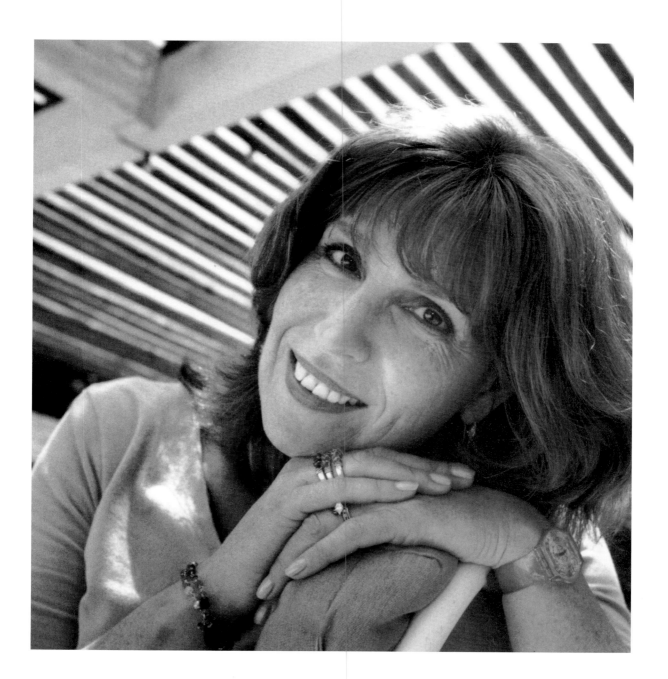

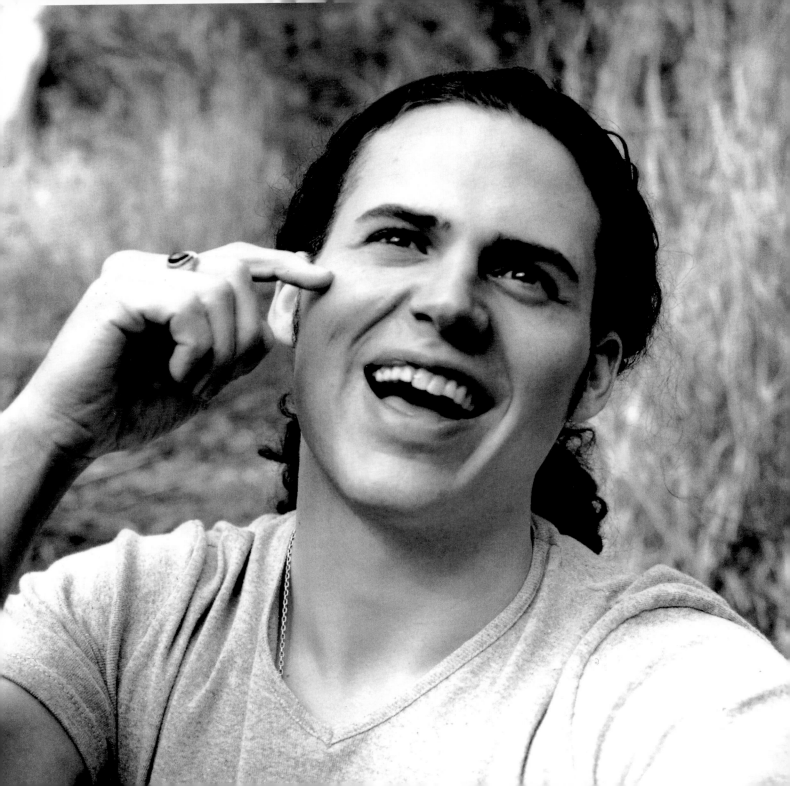

Bobby Davenport

ELEVEN-MONTH SURVIVOR
OSTEOSARCOMA

I WAS DIAGNOSED less than a year ago with osteosarcoma. The cancer hit my face; my maxilla—upper jaw—where the canine tooth would be. I had a little bump on my gum. I thought maybe I was kissing the wrong girl.

When the doctor said I had cancer I asked him if it was a good one and he said, "Oh, yes." I was joking around as a defense. It's what I do to get myself through trauma. I need time to let everything sink in. It's a talent I have for taking anything on. It helps me feel in control. I knew there was nothing I could do about my situation at that moment. When I walked to the elevator, a man stepped out and said hello in passing. I said hi in return, but what I wanted to say was, "Hi. I have cancer. Ten minutes ago I didn't know that I had cancer and now I do."

After the diagnosis I signed a paper agreeing that if they needed to, they could completely remove my maxilla and cheek, my lower eye lobe and eye, my upper eye lobe, and a portion of my forehead, back to my ear. If anything was left after that, I'd be extremely fortunate. But they were kind to me—they only took half my palate, part of my cheek and all of my upper left teeth.

Before the surgery I looked at my face. I told myself that I was beautiful, that I'd appreciated my face as much as I could until this point. Surgery was just around the corner. I either had to come to terms with it or get beat.

I was terrified during the initial few months because I didn't always know who I was. I had always associated myself with my business, with making money, with who I was dating, with my dog and with how my body looked. Those were the things that defined me and made me feel valuable. My cancer was a situation from which I could have profited or lost. I had every reason to feel sorry for myself, but the possibility of death gave me the opportunity to live life. That was something I hadn't done before.

I was planning on going through this by myself. I didn't know whether other people would want to hang out with me during this time. I'd left my family years before, and to have them back around me again—day in and day out—was overwhelming. The surgery was almost overshadowed by the fact that I was feeling love from them, and I began to recognize that nothing really mattered except living and the people who were there for me. And, hopefully, not losing half of my head.

I told my family that they were there to support me, that I came first and they come second; that I needed them to stay together. I wanted them to mimic my behavior. If I was acting strong, they needed to act strong. I told them that they would only hurt me if they started to cry. Anything too heavy would freak me out and affect my stability. I wanted them to set their feelings aside. I put pictures in my head of people I'd met and wondered how they would have handled my situation. I couldn't come up with anyone I wanted to model my behavior after but me. That was so freeing.

When I went to my first cancer support group to tell my story, I learned that if you say what you mean there will be consequences. I explained to the group that when I woke up from surgery I blinked each eye at least twenty-five times to double-check that I had both of them.

I pushed my fingers against my eyes, hard enough to cause discomfort. I wanted to be certain that they were there. I explained that I explored my face, hair-width by hair-width, until I recognized what was still there. I told everyone that I was laughing while I did it. The guy next to me in the group turned and started screaming "You want to see what it would look like if you lost your eye?" He pulled off his hat to show me where his eye had been. It was a nightmare. I didn't go back to the group for months. I knew I wasn't telling my story to hurt anyone or flaunt what I still had; I just wanted a turn to talk and say what I needed to say about my own experience.

I stopped radiation treatment about three and a half months ago. I've been really fatigued since then. I think it will take about six to twelve months for my energy to get back up again. I can do whatever I want, but there is always a consequence from it. For example, it took me days to recover from a run. Sometimes I feel that doctors think I'm feeling sorry for myself. They told me I was going to lose half my face and it was no big deal to them.

During radiation, I was manic in my drive. It was my way to cope. I own my own hardwood floor business and I run a crew of guys. Every day I would drive to work and I was dead tired. People would ask if I was feeling better yet. And the voices in my own head were asking if I was better, too. I was comparing myself to everyone else who was well and working.

Then I put myself on an "energy" schedule. Monday and Wednesday I would do a physical activity for an hour. One day on, one day off. I've also begun to meditate. Bad thoughts would come up and I'd try to blow them out of my mind. I'd pictured myself smiling and happy. Meditation settles me in a way I have never felt before.

Eventually I went back to the support group at Stanford and it's been easier since then. I think it's extremely important to be with others who have lived through this disease, but I still don't know how I feel about being a survivor. How do I figure it out? Can I say I'm cancer-free and that I will be my whole life? What if I get a recurrence? Is that going to crush me? What will happen to my foundation? My fear of recurrence is real. And it's scary. Especially when I meet people who are five and ten years cancer-free and then they relapse. The word *survivor* is a word that may or may not apply to me for a long time. But I don't think I'm ready to go yet. This has been my rebirth, and it's my time to share.

I recently went to a rave that was outside at a beautiful spot. The sun was coming up over the ocean and people were dancing. I really wanted to dance but I was scared to do it in front of so many people. Then I thought to myself, "You know what? I could only have this morning to really enjoy life." If I go to my doctor tomorrow, he could say the cancer is back. I learned through that realization that I'm not so worried about what others think of me anymore.

Recurrence scare, five months post-treatment

After radiation I began to have problems breathing through my nose. Polyps, which are mucous membrane growths, appeared in my sinus cavity. I did not go in to the doctor thinking that there was anything seriously wrong, but I was a little stressed because whenever I deal with someone who has the ability to take off the other half of my face, it's scary.

I'm supposed to snort salt water through my nostril every day to keep the cavity clean. But sometimes I don't do it because almost every time I do, it reminds me of having cancer. So I thought the doctor was going to tell me to keep it up; instead, he said I needed a biopsy. He said the word *biopsy* point-blank and that triggered everything for me. It was such a deep, shocking, shitty thing. It was as if somebody hit me and knocked me to the floor.

Suddenly, he was way up in my mouth with a big pair of scissors, and I was beginning to feel sick. When he finished, I was so worried and I felt anxiety and pain and guilt. I knew what I'd been through was painful, but he'd given me so much Novocaine that it didn't *really* hurt. Why did I feel that I'd underwent something so painful? I was trying to understand that what I was feeling was the word *biopsy* and all that it could mean again for me.

I didn't think I could go through another year of treatment with the same sort of positive, optimistic, I-can-handle-it attitude. I knew I couldn't do it again the same way I did the first time around. The idea of spending another eleven months alone in my apartment, cooking for myself and going through radiation again was just too much for me. The possibility that a tumor might have grown back while I was on treatment, that I might have to take chemotherapy and lose my hair and skin pigment again was rushing through my head. I told my girlfriend the news and was relieved when she said that she wanted to go through everything with me. She told me that I could be scared.

Later on that day, I drove down a beautiful road and I began to let myself think about the possibility of cancer returning. I thought about dying. I felt myself swelling with emotion. I was scared and angry and I started to cry. I was sure I had cancer again and I was trying to prepare myself.

Over the next few days I kept asking myself what I needed, what I wanted to do. I wanted to hike with my dog. I wanted to be outside. Then the doctor called. My biopsy was negative. When I heard the news, I felt such a release, it was as if I'd thrown up a sickness. I felt so alive again.

My girlfriend asked me once, during a difficult time, how much I could—at twenty-three—change. There are certain things that have helped me change incredibly: my first diagnosis, my spiritual awakening, certain treatments, and these three days in peril have changed me. I can let go of the old, I can become new. And after I heard the news, I felt new—again.

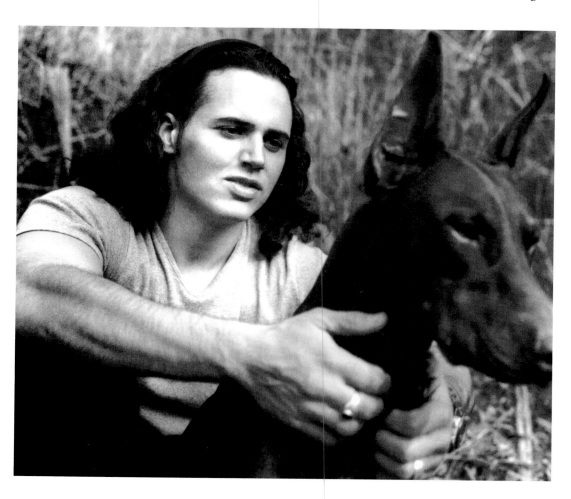

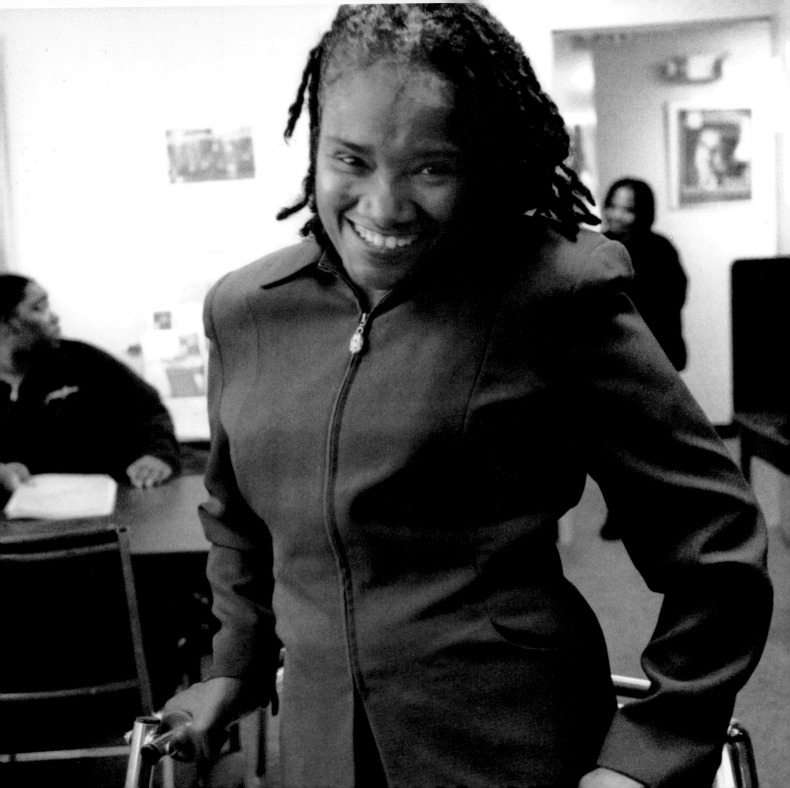

Diane Nero-Gaines

EIGHT-YEAR SURVIVOR
BREAST CANCER

I'M A QUADRIPLEGIC. Eight years ago, I was in Miami having physical therapy. While I was there, I noticed a large lump in my breast. The doctor said there was nothing wrong. I finished my therapy and came back to New York. Maybe two months later, I went to see my regular doctor and he examined me. The color went from his face. I had a mammogram and a needle aspiration. It was then I found out I had breast cancer.

The same week, the man I had lived with for fifteen years died of complications from diabetes. I had to schedule my surgery and bury my daughters' father at the same time. I just wanted to wake up from the bad dream. I truly believe the human brain has a safety switch that automatically switches off. I became numb.

I knew I had to take care of my girls. At that time, my daughters were sixteen, twenty-one, and twenty-two. I had to reassure them that I wasn't going to die, even though, inside, I didn't believe it. Before I went into the hospital for my mastectomy, I felt like I was looking at everything for the last time, but I didn't tell anyone. I couldn't put that on anybody.

The doctors said I came through the surgery with flying colors, but I was in such pain, and every time I sat up I felt like I was going to pass out or throw up. I had a bad reaction to the dye for some tests and I got lockjaw, and at that point I decided I couldn't take any more. I wasn't eating and I just lay there. I was giving up, and that scared me 'cause I don't give up. But my friend Becky put me in my wheelchair, rolled me into the sunroom at the hospital, and told me all the reasons I had to live. She told me that I had to use the challenges; that I was a fighter, that I had to reach down inside and pull out whatever strength I had left. I promised her I would, and from that day on I thought I was going to live.

A couple of months later, I started chemotherapy. I was supposed to have six treatments. By the third one, my hands and tongue had black spots, my skin color changed and all my nails turned black. I would drag myself into the office and just put my head on the desk. I felt like a walking dead person. And I said, "I can't do this." I wanted somebody to give me permission to stop the chemotherapy.

After the fourth treatment, I made the decision not to go back. Everyone begged me not to: my brother, my girls, the oncologist and the nurses—they were very upset with me. But I had to make the decision between the quantity of my life or the quality. I just couldn't take it anymore. When I left that office, I felt that I had gotten my life back.

The decision to quit chemo was the hardest decision I'd ever made in my life. I felt I wasn't giving myself a chance; like I was deciding to die because I wasn't doing what the doctors said I should do. I thought, why did I even bother in the first place if I wasn't even going to see it through? I owed it to my family to do whatever I could to live, but the chemo was killing me. I just made the decision that I was going to start living my life. I didn't know how long it was going to be, but I realized that I had always been Diane Worry Gaines. I had to control everything and take care of everybody—I came last. Not this time. I began to feel so happy; it was like I'd gotten a new lease on life.

Everything began to matter to me, all the good things. The birds had been singing all the years of my life but I had never heard them. I was getting in touch with the universe and I never questioned my decision after that. I told myself that I was going to make great memories, no matter how much time I had. I took every dime I'd ever saved and took my family to the Bahamas. We had never traveled and we had a ball. It opened up a whole new world for my daughters, and they have been traveling ever since.

Never before cancer would I have spent the money to go to the places I've been since. I just went on a little cruise to Norway, and I just bought a time-share for my grandkids. I was able to plan my daughter's wedding. Watching my grandchildren grow up has given me the years chemo took away. I thank God every day I'm alive to see them. So if I didn't know how to live life before, I'm living it now. I have no complaints.

A few years ago I went to a party and met a man from Barbados. We're good friends and, since that time, I go there twice a year. That's my retreat. I chill and rejuvenate, eat good food. I've grown emotionally during those trips; I have a lot of time to myself with unfinished business. Sometimes I still hold up too tight. In our family we were always taught to be strong. My maiden name is Merrill, and I always heard, "If you're a Merrill, you can take anything." Crying was a weakness. But when I am away, I am able to cry, to feel what I need to feel and let it go.

At twenty-four I suffered a spinal cord injury. When I first became physically challenged, I knew I wouldn't be able to do the things I'd done before. So I went back to school and I ended up getting a master's degree in criminal justice. Now I'm program director for a community

I love people and I love working with them. But sometimes I don't want to hear the words breast cancer, and I have to back away from the group. Then I'm like, Diane, you have to give back, and I go and I'm glad I'm at the meetings. But I'm not Diane Breast Cancer Gaines. Sometimes I just want to go see a funny movie.

corrections program that is an alternative to incarceration for female offenders. The population I work with has to overcome a lot of challenges. A lot of them know what I've been through and they think, "God, if she can go through that I know I can do what I have to do." I don't see myself as amazing, or whatever adjective people use, but I do what I have to and I love life. I'm not the kind of person to lie around and vegetate.

I had joined a cancer support group when I was on chemo. There were about eight Caucasian woman and three African-American women. We all connected, but there was something missing. Our issues were different. African-Americans don't have a lot of the information others have. Whites are pretty knowledgeable about this disease. They receive good care and service from doctors, but I don't think African-Americans get the same education and treatment—we're on our own. I was very fortunate that I had white women friends who had been through this and could guide me. I helped start another group for African-American women that I still go to. I love that group. The women were so supportive, and it helped me get over the shame that I had around cancer.

I love people and I love working with them. But sometimes I don't want to hear the words *breast cancer*, and I have to back away from the group. Then I'm like, Diane, you have to give back, and I go and I'm glad I'm at the meetings. But I'm not Diane Breast Cancer Gaines. Sometimes I just want to go see a funny movie.

In the beginning, when I became physically challenged, I wasn't empowered—I was lost. I wanted to give up so many times but I didn't. I reached inside and pulled out everything that was needed to go on. I tried to do the same with cancer.

In life, so many people have gotten the short end of the stick. You just need somebody to turn that around to see there's so much more. I used to love to dance. I loved going to parties and hearing the music. Sometimes, when I close my eyes, I'm dancing.

Resources

∎

MANY WORTHY ORGANIZATIONS are devoted to helping people with cancer, including several groups that were founded by people profiled in this book. The following list provides contact information for those organizations, as well as other groups that those in this book found to be particularly helpful.

THE KEVIN HEARN FUND
Princess Margaret Hospital Foundation
610 University Ave.
Toronto, Ontario M5G 2M9
Canada
Telephone: (416) 946-6560

> *Proceeds of the Kevin Hearn Fund benefit bone marrow transplant and leukemia treatment research.*

CANADIAN CANCER SOCIETY
National Office
10 Alcorn Avenue, Suite 200
Toronto, Ontario M4V 3B1
Telephone: (416) 961-7223
www.cancer.ca

THE ERIC DAVIS FOUNDATION
c/o Angela Hunt
Celebrity Images, Inc.
22 Ingate Terrace
Baltimore, MD 21277
Telephone: (410) 536-8149

> *Raising awareness and funding research to help improve prevention and screening techniques, and to find new treatments for colorectal cancer. Also, The Eric Davis Foundation is a sponsor of the Score Against Colon Cancer campaign, which educates the general public about the importance of getting tested early for colorectal cancer: (877) SCORE-123*

CANCERVIVE

11636 Chayote St.
Los Angeles, CA 90049
Telephone: (800) 4-TO-CURE
  or (310) 203-9232
www.cancervive.org

The mission of Cancervive is to assist those who have experienced cancer to assimilate the physical, emotional and psychosocial changes brought about by the illness. Cancervive provides services and educational materials for cancer patients, survivors and family members as they deal with the aftermath of the disease.

YEARS TO YOUR LIFE HEALTH CENTER

237 W. Page
Dallas, Texas 75208
Telephone: (214) 339-0066

Colon irrigation and nutritional consulting.

ULMAN CANCER FUND FOR YOUNG ADULTS

PMB 505
4725 Dorsey Hall Drive, Suite A
Ellicott City, MD 21402
Telephone: (410) 964-0202
www.ulmanfund.org

To provide support programs, education and resources, free of charge, to benefit young adults, their families and friends, who are affected by cancer, and to promote awareness and prevention of cancer.

LANCE ARMSTRONG FOUNDATION

P.O. Box 161150
Austin, TX 78716-1150
Telephone: (512) 236-8820
www.laf.org

The Lance Armstrong Foundation helps cancer patients of all ages through medical and scientific research grants, development of after-treatment services and support for survivors, public education and awareness programs, and information and support to those diagnosed with cancer.

THE BREAST CANCER FUND

2107 O'Farrell Street
San Francisco, CA 94115
Telephone: (415) 346-8223
www.breastcancerfund.org

The Breast Cancer Fund aims to end breast cancer through public education, advocacy, patient support initiatives and research. Every initiative, from mountain climbs to art exhibits, makes an effort to change the way people think about breast cancer from personal tragedy to public health crisis, and to promote an approach to wellness and healing that encompasses the mind, body and spirit of every woman.

THE WELLNESS COMMUNITY

530 Hampshire Road
Westlake Village, CA 91361
Telephone: (805) 379-4777
  and
1320 Centre Street, Suite 305
Newton Centre, MA 02159-2444
Telephone: (617) 332-1919

The mission of the Wellness Community is to help people with cancer fight for their recovery by providing free psychological and emotional support as an adjunct to conventional medical treatment. There are 19 Wellness Communities in various locations across the United States.

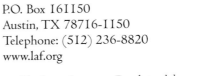

THE LEUKEMIA & LYMPHOMA SOCIETY, INC.
1311 Mamaroneck Ave.
White Plains, NY, 10605
Telephone: (914) 949-5213
www.leukemia-lymphoma.org

The Leukemia & Lymphoma Society's mission is to cure leukemia, lymphoma, Hodgkin's disease and myeloma, and to improve the quality of life of patients and their families. The Leukemia and Lymphoma Society also sponsors Team in Training (www.teamintraining.org), the largest endurance training program in the United States. Participants raise money toward a cure for leukemia and lymphoma in exchange for coaching, training, and travel opportunities to participate in a marathon, century bicycle ride, or triathlon.

SISTERS' NETWORK
National Headquarters
8787 Woodway Drive—Suite 4206
Houston, TX 77063
Telephone: (713) 781-0255
www.sistersnetworkinc.org

Sisters' Network is committed to increasing local and national attention to the devastating impact that breast cancer has in the African-American Community.

PLANET CANCER
1804 E. 39th St.
Austin, Texas 78722
Telephone: (512) 481-9010
www.planetcancer.org

Planet Cancer brings young adults with cancer together to provide each other with emotional support, understanding, and information, creating a peer network where they can freely express thoughts, fears, attitudes, and insights that are particularly relevant to young adulthood.

THE AMERICAN CANCER SOCIETY
National Headquarters
American Cancer Society
1599 Clifton Road
Atlanta, GA 30329
Telephone: 1-800-ACS-2345
www.cancer.org

HODGKIN'S DISEASE MAIL LIST
www.hodgkinsdisease.org

An Internet mailing list dedicated to the exchange of information concerning Hodgkin's Disease.

THE SADICK FAMILY FUND FOR UROLOGY RESEARCH
NYU Medical Center, Office of Development
316 East 30th Street
New York, NY 10016

The Sadick Family Fund was established in honor of Dr. Victor Nitti and Dr. Samir Taneja, Barbara Sadick's surgeons. Proceeds go to fund urology research.